AP

SI

WITHDRAWN
UTSA LIBRARIES

D1443067

Corporate Violence

CORPORATE VIOLENCE

Injury and Death for Profit

EDITED BY

Stuart L. Hills

Rowman & Littlefield
PUBLISHERS

ROWMAN & LITTLEFIELD

Published in the United States of America in 1987
by Rowman & Littlefield, Publishers
(a division of Littlefield, Adams & Company)
81 Adams Drive, Totowa, New Jersey 07512

Copyright © 1987 by Rowman & Littlefield

All rights reserved. No part of this publication may
be reproduced, stored in a retrieval system, or transmitted
in any form or by any means, electronic, mechanical,
photocopying, recording, or otherwise, without the prior
permission of the publisher.

Library of Congress Cataloging-in-Publication Data

Corporate violence.

Includes bibliographies.   Index.
1. Corporations—Corrupt practices. 2. Corporate
profits—moral and ethical aspects. 3. Health risk
assessment. 4. Commercial crime.
I. Hills, Stuart L.
HG4028.P7C67   1986   363.1'1   86-22119
ISBN 0-8476-7535-1
ISBN 0-8476-7536-X (pbk.)

89 88 87
6 5 4 3 2 1

Printed in the United States of America

LIBRARY
The University of Texas
At San Antonio

Contents

Preface

THIS ANTHOLOGY focuses on *corporate violence:* actual harm and risk of harm inflicted on consumers, workers, and the general public as a result of decisions by corporate executives or managers, from corporate negligence, the quest for profits at any cost, and willful violations of health, safety, and environmental laws. In the last two decades, there has been a growing public concern about reports of exploding automobiles, defective medical devices, inadequately tested drugs, and other hazardous products that are manufactured and marketed despite knowledge by corporate officials that such products can injure and kill consumers. There are reports of toxic chemical dumps that have poisoned drinking supplies, caused leukemia in children, and destroyed entire communities; of cover-ups of asbestos-induced cancer, and the gradual suffocation of workers from inhaling cotton dust; of radioactive water leaking from improperly maintained nuclear reactors; of mangled bodies and lives snuffed out in unsafe coal mines and steel mills—and other dangers to our health and safety.

Yet, public understanding of corporate violence is vague, obscured by crime statistics and the preoccupation of law enforcement officials and the public with violent street crimes reinforcing the popular belief that harmful, illegal acts are perpetrated mainly by the pathological, the poor, and the powerless. I hope, in this brief anthology, to heighten awareness of the vast scope of serious harm caused by the illegal acts of "respectable" business executives who impersonally kill and maim many more Americans than street muggers and assailants. These highly publicized, conventional street crimes, however, still evoke the most immediate fear in the public, command the largest share of our law enforcement resources, and more importantly, divert attention from the crimes of the privileged and powerful groups in America.

The Introduction to this anthology provides a brief overview of the nature of corporate violence, the magnitude of the threat to the safety and health of the general public, and the growing awareness of the importance of this pattern of corporate crime. The articles in Parts I, II, and III are intended to reveal more clearly the kinds and extent of injuries inflicted on consumers and workers, and the impact of

vii

corporate violence on the lives of real people in their neighborhoods and communities. In Part IV, "Voices from the Corporate Bureaucracy," personal accounts of the experiences of corporate employees, whistle-blowers, and middle-managers reveal the flexible moralities and corporate pressures that engulf many business executives, and lead some of them to violate the law and their own ethical principles.

In the Epilogue, I highlight characteristic patterns of corporate violence, with particular emphasis on the organizational strains on business executives and the rationalizations provided by the corporate subculture to neutralize feelings of guilt. The Epilogue explores the ways in which impersonal corporations diffuse responsibility and foster an ethical insensitivity that can result in grave injuries despite the fact that none of the corporate offenders may have intended to cause any harm to the victims. Indeed, because the pursuit of profit is a worthy goal in our society, and corporate managers are pressured to make decisions for "the good of the company," bureaucrats frequently become indifferent to issues of health and safety. Consequently, corporate violence can take on a certain banality that cannot be explained by theories applicable to individual predatory street crimes.

To maintain the interest of undergraduate students, I have selected articles that are highly readable, stimulating, and insightful in their presentation of the nature of corporate violence. Although the anthology is designed primarily for supplementary reading in college courses in criminology, social deviance, social problems, and business and society, I hope the book will prove useful to a wider audience: encouraging both the student reader and the general public to explore more deeply the study of this complex pattern of violence, and raising the critical questions that will help create a more humane society. To help the interested reader and to encourage further inquiry, I've provided a list of additional readings at the end of each section.

This book was completed during my sabbatical leave, and I am grateful to St. Lawrence University for providing me with financial support and this opportunity. I am also deeply grateful to Mary Haught and Jean Deese who typed most of the manuscript, and to David Friedrichs, Martin Schwartz, Ronald Kramer, and David Simon for their support and constructive comments on this project.

Acknowledgments

Grateful acknowledgment is made to the authors and publishers who have granted permission to reprint the following selections.

"Pinto Madness" by Mark Dowie from *Mother Jones* 2 (September/October 1977), pp. 18–32. Reprinted by permission of the author.

"At Any Cost: Corporate Greed, Women, and the Dalkon Shield" by Morton Mintz from *The Progressive* 49 (November 1985), pp. 20–25. From the book *At Any Cost: Corporate Greed, Women, and the Dalkon Shield* by Morton Mintz. Copyright © 1985 by Morton Mintz. Reprinted by permission of Pantheon Books, a Division of Random House, Inc., New York, N.Y.

"The Dumping of Hazardous Products on Foreign Markets" by Mark Dowie and *Mother Jones* from *Mother Jones* 4 (November 1979), pp. 23–44. Reprinted by permission of Mark Dowie and *Mother Jones*.

"The Invisible Risk" by Mark Reutter from *Mother Jones* 5 (August 1980), pp. 49–60. Reprinted by permission of *Mother Jones*.

"Death by Cotton Dust" by Richard Guarasci. An original article prepared for this book.

"Manslaughter in a Coal Mine" by Harry M. Caudill from *The Nation* 224 (April 23, 1977), pp. 492–97. Reprinted by permission of The Nation Magazine/Nation Associates Inc. 1977.

"Murder in the Workplace" by Nancy Frank from *Crimes Against Health and Safety*. Copyright © 1985 by Nancy Frank. Reprinted by permission of Harrow and Heston, Publishers.

"Chemical Dumping as a Corporate Way of Life" by Matt Tallmer from *The Progressive* 45 (November 1981), pp. 35–42. Copyright © 1981, The Progressive, Inc. Reprinted by permission of The Progressive, Madison, Wis.

"A Slap on the Wrist for the Kepone Mob" by Christopher D. Stone from *Business and Society Review* (Summer 1977), pp. 4–11. Copyright © 1977 by Warren, Gorham, & Lamont, Inc. Reprinted with permission of Warren, Gorham, and Lamont.

"Who's Burning Boston?" by James P. Brady from "Arson, Fiscal Crisis, and Community Action," *Crime and Delinquency* 28 (April 1982), pp. 249–61. Copyright 1982 by the National Council on Crime and Delinquency. Reprinted by permission of Sage Publications, Inc., Beverly Hills, Calif.

"Why Should My Conscience Bother Me?" by Kermit Vandivier from *In the Name of Profit* by Robert L. Heilbroner. Copyright © 1972 by Doubleday & Company, Inc., New York, N.Y. Reprinted by permission of the publisher.

"Benton Harlow: Distributor of Unsafe Drugs" by James T. Carey from James T. Carey, *Introduction to Criminology,* © 1978, pp. 379–86. Reprinted by permission of Prentice-Hall, Englewood Cliffs, New Jersey.

"Exposing Risks of Nuclear Disaster: Confessions of a Whistle Blower" by Peter Faulkner from Alan F. Westin, ed., *Whistle Blowing!* © 1981 Educational Fund for Individual Rights. Reprinted by permission of McGraw-Hill Book Company.

Introduction

On March 14, 1976, a front-page story in the *Washington Star* reported a coal mine explosion with the headline: "Mine is Closed 26 Deaths Late." The news article raised a number of serious questions about the safety of the mine:

Why, the relatives [of the 26 dead miners] ask, did the mine ventilation fail and allow pockets of volatile methane gas to build up in a shaft 2,300 feet below the surface?

Why wasn't the mine cleared as soon as supervisors spotted evidence of methane gas near where miners were driving hugh machines into the 61-foot-high coal seam? . . .

In Washington, Sen. Harrison Williams, D–NJ, said investigators of the Senate Labor and Welfare Committee which he chairs have found that there have been 1,250 safety violations at the 13-year-old mine since 1970. Fifty-seven of those violations were serious enough for federal inspectors to order the mine closed and 21 of those were in cases where federal inspectors felt there was imminent danger to the lives of the miners working there, he said. . . .

Federal inspectors said the most recent violations found at the mine were three found in the ventilation system on Monday—the day before 15 miners were killed.[1]

On the same page was another news story with the headline: "Mass Murder Claims Six in Pennsylvania." The article told of a suburban Philadelphia family, a father, mother, and three children, shot to death. Yet, why do news stories refer to mass murder or homicide, in this instance, but typically, in cases such as mine explosions, refer to "accidents," "tragic disaster," "acts of God" or "uncontrollable forces of nature"? Why aren't operators of the coal company charged with reckless mass homicide or criminally negligent manslaughter? Although in such work settings there is no deliberate intent to kill the miners, the mine operators may *willfully* and *knowingly* intend to violate the safety regulations in order to reduce operating costs and increase profits, aware that such decisions place the lives of their workers in jeopardy. In the case of the Philadelphia family, we realize that the violence affects real people, its source is obvious, the action is clearly criminal; in the case of the mine explosion, it is not apparent that the deaths and injuries are caused by real persons in respectable

1

positions of responsibility within a corporate bureaucracy. However, both actions, one direct, the other remote and fragmented, result in deaths to their victims.

Deaths in American coal mines have long been accepted as the "price of doing dangerous work." Yet there is compelling evidence that the vast majority of such deaths are preventable. In England, which has the safest coal mining industry in the world, the fatality rate per worker-hour is only one-third of that in the United States, even though the geological conditions for mining in England are, in fact, much more dangerous. Moreover, in the United States there is considerable variability in death rates among different mining companies and during different periods of time. For example, the United States Steel Corporation does not have a fatalistic resignation toward deaths, nor does it place a low priority on safety (attitudes once typical of most of the coal industry); in this company, safety precautions and compliance with regulatory laws are the responsibility of top management. Consequently, accident and death rates in mines operated by U.S. Steel are among the lowest in the coal industry.[2]

In the 1970s, technological advances combined with new safety legislation and more frequent inspection helped to bring about a significant decline in mining fatalities. In the early 1980s however, the political mood changed as the newly elected administration campaigned on a deregulatory platform to "get the government off our backs." Federal spending on mine health and safety inspection declined sharply and deaths in the coal mines once again began to mount.[3]

In large measure, conceptions of social reality reflect the culture and structure of a society—its traditions, conventional beliefs, media images, and dominant economic and political institutions. As Michael Harrington points out, "most people see only what their times and culture permit them to see."[4] In America, a deeply ingrained *individualistic bias* in our criminal justice system often makes it difficult to label physical harm caused by the actions of business organizations "violence."

From "Hill Street Blues" to the shoot-outs in "Miami Vice," the media bombard us daily with reports of street violence—individual killings, muggings, assaults, and rapes. Although in the last two decades the news media have increased their coverage of corporate wrongdoing, especially in cases with dramatic impact, the mass media still typically attribute instances of physical harm to consumers or the public to "tragic accidents," "technical errors," or "faulty judgment." Corporate practices that injure and kill consumers, or cause slow-to-develop crippling diseases among industrial workers become problems of "product liability" and are reported as "business news."

Occasionally, reporters label a corporate polluter an "industry renegade," or pinpoint the individual greed of a particular business official as the locus of the problem.

Yet, in a capitalistic economy where business is oriented to profit-making, the possibility that corporate *organizational* goals and priorities might *systematically* generate life-threatening situations as a byproduct of standard operating procedures gets short shift in the popular media. Instead, the public is more likely to witness corporate denials and stone-walling, regulatory agency warnings, "cease-and-desist" orders, contested product recalls, government-financed pollution clean-ups, miniscule civil fines levied on multibillion dollar corporations, or out-of-court settlements. Criminal convictions are infrequent, and rarely do corporate offenders languish in prison.

In a business-for-profit economy, governmental intervention in "free enterprise" has often been suspect or actively resisted. This attitude has been reinforced in the 1980s by the Reagan administration's support of laissez-faire ideology. In a nation where the prevailing view has traditionally been that "business is business," not crime, many Americans seem to alternate between shock and outrage at the latest exposé of corporate wrongdoing, and cynical resignation that, when it comes to "making a buck," anything goes. In any case, few Americans comprehend the prevalence and far-reaching consequences of corporate violence in this country.

According to the FBI *Uniform Crime Reports,* in 1985 there were roughly 19,000 murders and nonnegligent manslaughters, and 723,000 reported cases of aggravated assault. Yet the National Safety Council has reported that work-related accidents alone have caused some 13,000 deaths annually and 2.2 million disabling work injuries. Government studies have estimated that the annual number of deaths from all occupationally related causes is probably over 100,000, the majority of which many researchers attribute to company negligence or willful disregard of government health and safety laws.[5] Most occupational deaths result from disease (such as job-related cancer and respiratory ailments) and therefore are the result of conditions beyond the control of workers:

> Examples of such conditions are the level of coal dust in the air (about 10 percent of all active coal miners have black lung disease), or textile dust (some 85,000 American cotton textile workers presently suffer breathing impairments due to acute byssinosis or brown lung, and another 35,000 former mill workers are totally disabled with chronic brown lung), or asbestos fibers (a study of 632 asbestos-insulation workers between 1943 and 1971 indicates that 11 percent have died of asbestosis and 38 percent of cancer . . .), or coal tars ("workers who had been employed five or more years in the coke

ovens died of lung cancer at a rate of three and a half times that for all steel workers"; coke oven workers also develop cancer of the scrotum at a rate five times that of the general population). Also some 800,000 people suffer from occupationally related skin disease each year . . . and "the number of American workers experiencing noise conditions that may damage their hearing is estimated . . . to be in excess of 6 million, and may even reach 16 million."[6]

Not only in the workplace are citizens at risk from corporate violence. The National Commission on Product Safety has estimated that there are approximately 20 million serious injuries annually associated with consumer products. As several articles in this anthology make clear, the sale of defective automobiles, appliances, and medical devices, the consumption of unsafe food and drugs, and the use of other hazardous consumer products result in an estimated 100,000 permanently disabled persons and 30,000 deaths each year.[7]

Entire communities are at peril. For example New York's Love Canal and Times Beach, Missouri, are threatened with destruction from toxic chemical waste dumps. Homes must be abandoned and anguished parents watch their children, some with serious birth defects, fearing signs of developing cancer from having played in contaminated soil.[8] And in cities like Boston and New York, arson-for-profit schemes destroy entire neighborhoods, often with the complicity of respectable officials in real estate, insurance, banking, and government agencies.[9]

[Clearly, corporate crime destroys, injures, and kills many more victims than media headlines and crime statistics would lead us to believe.] Ronald Kramer provides a useful definition of corporate violence:

Corporate violence is corporate behavior which produces an unreasonable risk of physical harm to employees, the general public, and consumers, which is the result of deliberate decision-making by persons who occupy positions as corporation managers or executives, which is organizationally based, and which is intended to benefit the corporation itself.[10]

[But investigations of corporate violence must reach beyond violations of the criminal law, since few corporate offenders are dealt with in criminal courts—one of the privileges of power and social status in America. Gigantic corporations have the wealth, legal expertise, and organizational clout to help shape both the laws and the kinds of legal settings in which their socially injurious behavior is handled (including sometimes the power to keep their harmful actions even from being defined as illegal).[Corporate offenders are much more likely to be tacitly sanctioned in *civil* courts or by quasi-judicial *regulatory*

agencies like the Food and Drug Administration, Occupational Safety and Health Administration, and the Environmental Protection Administration. Biases favoring large corporations are so deeply ingrained in the American culture and political structure that the legal profession is not aware of the discrimination that exists against individuals. We simply do not see corporate crime as crime. For research purposes, therefore, corporate violence should include any physically injurious act that could be punished by the government, regardless of whether the corporate offense is punishable under civil, administrative, or criminal law. As Clinard and Yeager contend:

> Unless this more inclusive definition of crime is used, it is not possible to consider violations of law by corporations in the same context as ordinary crime. In legal terms, business and corporate offenders are "administratively segregated" from ordinary offenders not because of differences in illegal actions but because of differences in legal terminology.[11]

In America, there is growing concern with corporate decision-making that is indifferent to human lives and suffering. The following examples are the result of such decision-making: the decision to continue to sell the deadly Ford Pinto and defective Firestone 500 radial tires;[12] the midnight dumping of poisonous wastes;[13] the cover-ups by Johns-Manville officials and company doctors of the hazards of working with asbestos, thereby subjecting thousands of workers to slow and painful deaths from cancer;[14] the Three Mile Island nuclear reactor disaster;[15] the horribly deformed thalidomide babies;[16] the manufacturing of defective airplanes and cutbacks in airline maintenance[17]; and other hazards to life and limb brought on in large measure by corporate negligence, the quest for profits, and deliberate violations of health, safety, and environmental laws. Although public awareness is still fragmented and unfocused, popular films such as "The China Syndrome" and "Silkwood," investigative news programs like "60 Minutes," the growing consumer and environmental movements, and attempts to dismantle or weaken regulatory agencies such as the EPA and OSHA,[18] have helped alert many Americans to the threat from "crime in the suites." Yet, as Kramer points out, "the victims of this corporate violence remain invisible for the most part. Our society refuses to see them."[19] It is the purpose of this anthology to help the reader see more clearly the faces of these victims, to make them and their suffering more visible.

Recent empirical studies have documented the seriousness with which the general public regards corporate acts that cause physical injury. These studies also show clearly that the public supports more severe penalties for harmful behavior than are currently imposed by most court judges and regulatory agencies.[20] Nevertheless, preoccupation of the media and law enforcement agencies with conventional crimes committed by the poor and powerless limits public understanding of the range and magnitude of corporate violence. For instance, few Americans are probably aware that unsafe drugs, toxic pesticides, defective contraceptive devices, and carcinogens banned in this country have been routinely dumped on Third World countries where health and safety laws are less stringent or nonexistent. In what Mark Dowie calls the "corporate crime of the century," multinational corporations have failed to warn physicians and consumers in other countries of the full range of dangerous side effects and hazardous risks involved.[21]

Consider, for example, the Dalkon Shield intrauterine device for birth control. U.S. District Judge Miles Lord, who presided over a court settlement of seven "product liability" cases, accused top executives of the A.H. Robins Company of putting profits above the health of women and causing "catastrophic harm" to women who used this IUD. In a dramatic courtroom scene, Lord described the Dalkon Shield as "an instrument of death, mutilation and disease" by which thousands of users had become infertile, had involuntary abortions, or developed pelvic inflammatory disease. After seventeen women died, the Robins Company finally took the Dalkon Shield off the market in the face of massive lawsuits and pressure from the Food and Drug Administration, but continued to export millions of unsterilized IUDs overseas, still marketing them as "modern, superior and safe."[22]

In a global economy with worldwide markets, the potential impact of hazardous corporate activities is enormous. According to Dowie, at least five manufacturers have exported 450,000 baby pacifiers of the type that have caused infants to choke to death after the Consumer Product Safety Commission (CPSC) proposed a ban on their sale. And one can only venture a guess as to how many children have developed cancer from the several million garments coated with the fire retardant chemical Tris, shipped to other countries after the CPSC ordered the carcinogenic chemical off the American market.[23]

Probably few Americans are also aware that in the worst nuclear disaster in American history—the highly publicized near melt-down at Three Mile Island—the operators of the plant, Metropolitan Edison, falsified test data on water leaking from the reactor's primary cooling system for at least five months prior to the accident. According to Nuclear Regulatory Commission officials, the attempt to avoid a shut-down of the reactor plant by faking safety tests could have contributed to the seriousness of the accident. Convicted of falsifying records, an action that endangered the lives of thousands of people in the area, Metropolitan Edison agreed to pay a paltry $45,000 fine in a plea bargain in which the utility pleaded guilty to one count and *nolo contendere* (no contest) to six other charges.[24]

While many news readers have learned of the defective Ford Pinto automobile, it is unlikely that they are aware of the internal Ford memorandum that revealed the callous indifference to human life and suffering. When Ford engineers discovered that the fuel tank on the Pinto ruptured upon rear-end impact at speeds as low as 25 miles per hour—exploding into flames from any spark of scraping metal—company executives ordered a cost-benefit analysis on the problem. Projecting millions of car sales, Ford decided it was not worth making an $11 alteration per car to save several hundred lives, and for seven years continued to manufacture and sell a car they knew could become a rolling incinerator.[25]

Ford, of course, is not the only automobile manufacture to engage in corporate violence against consumers. In 1983, the Justice Department filed a criminal action against General Motors for deliberately concealing problems with its front-wheel-drive 1980 X-cars. Documents released in another civil suit against GM revealed that test drivers and internal company documents repeatedly warned key company executives just prior to general production that the rear wheel brakes had a tendency to lock prematurely, causing the car to spin dangerously out of control. Despite more than 1,700 complaints, and at least 71 known injuries and 15 deaths, GM has bitterly fought the government's attempt to force a recall to repair, without any charge to the owners, of over one million 1980 X-cars.[26]

Sociologists do not yet fully understand all of the complex causes of corporate violence. Since Edwin Sutherland's pioneering work on corporate crime, published in 1949, social scientists have conducted only a handful of in-depth empirical studies of corporate violence. A number of unresolved empirical and theoretical questions remain before we can adequately explain and more effectively control corporate acts that injure and kill:

> We need, for example, to develop an understanding of the political economy of corporate violence; we need to know how and why a corporate capitalist economy systematically generates such violence, and why the state in a capitalist society is so impotent in its attempts to control these acts. We need also to understand how organizational environments, goals, and structures relate to corporate violence.[27]

As Robert Jackall notes, we also need "to understand how bureaucracy separates men and women from the consequences of their actions" and how "such depersonalization reinforces the avoidance of responsibility."[28] While an examination of all of these crucial questions is beyond the scope of this brief anthology, in the Epilogue I explore some of the organizational conditions in a large business corporation that may contribute to decisions that have life-threatening consequences. The study of corporate violence provides important opportunities for sociologists to better understand the ways in which complex hierarchical organizations routinely foster a pragmatic structural amorality—an ethical numbness—that can bring immense human suffering to others.

In a capitalistic economy dominated by multinational corporations where the profit motive is supreme, where decentralized decision-making diffuses responsibility, where the quest for economic success and security are managerial imperatives, and where a company engineer or corporate manager is more absorbed by the constraints of carrying out his or her specific tasks than by the probable results of those tasks, evil takes on a certain *banality*. As I shall explore further in the Epilogue, this apparent indifference to ultimate consequences, to faceless victims, may well be the "greater cause of avoidable human suffering" inflicted by large-scale corporations rather than intent to harm.[29]

NOTES

1. Quoted in Jeffrey H. Reiman, *The Rich Get Richer and the Poor Get Prison* (New York: Wiley, 1984), p. 35.

2. John Braithwaite, *To Punish or Persuade: Enforcement of Coal Mine Safety* (Albany: State University of New York Press, 1985), pp. 10, 42.

3. Ibid., p. 81; Lorin E. Kerr, James L. Weeks, and Maier B. Fox, "Reckless Deregulation in the Coal Mines," *Business and Society Review* (Winter 1983), pp. 52–57; "Death in the Darkness," *Time* 1 March 1982, pp. 18–19.

4. Michael Harrington, *Decade of Decision: The Crisis of the American System* (New York: Simon and Schuster, 1980), p. 222.

5. Reiman, pp. 52–53; Raymond J. Michalowski, *Order, Law, and Crime* (New York: Random, 1985), pp. 325, 328.

6. Reiman, pp. 56–67.

7. Laura S. Schrager and James P. Short, Jr., "Toward a Sociology of Organizational Crime," *Social Problems* 25 (June 1978), p. 415.

8. Michael H. Brown, *Laying Waste: The Poisoning of America by Toxic Chemicals* (New York: Pantheon, 1980); Tracy Freedman and David Weir, "Polluting the Most Vulnerable," *The Nation*, 236 (14 May 1983), pp. 600–604; E. R. Shipp, "Only 2 Remain in Dioxin Ghost Town," *The New York Times*, 8 April 1986, p. A–20.

9. James Brady, "Arson, Fiscal Crisis, and Community Action," *Crime and Delinquency* 28 (April 1982), pp. 247–70; an abridged version of this article is reprinted in this anthology under the title "Who's Burning Boston?"

10. Ronald C. Kramer, "A Prolegomenon to the Study of Corporate Violence," *Humanity and Society* 7 (May 1983), p. 166.

11. Marshall B. Clinard and Peter C. Yeager, *Corporate Crime* (New York: The Free Press, 1980), p. 16.

12. Lee Patrick Strobel, *Reckless Homicide? Ford's Pinto Trial* (South Bend, Ind.: And Books, 1980); U.S. Department of Transportation, *Firestone Fined $500,000 for Tire Safety Violations* (Washington, D.C.: Department of Transportation Office of Public Affairs, 1980).

13. Alan A. Block and Frank R. Scarpitti, *Poisoning for Profit* (New York: Morrow, 1985).

14. Paul Brodeur, *Outrageous Misconduct: The Asbestos Industry on Trial* (New York: Pantheon, 1985); Samuel S. Epstein, *The Politics of Cancer* (San Francisco: Sierra Club, 1978), pp. 83–100.

15. "Met-Ed Admits Falsifying TMI Test Records," *Syracuse Post–Dispatch*, 29 February 1984, p. 1; "Faking it at 3 Mile Island?" *The New York Times*, 12 November 1983, p. 8–E. For reports of safety violations and problems at other nuclear facilities, see also Dennis Bernstein and Connie Blitt, "Lethal Dose," *The Progressive* 50 (March 1986), pp. 22–25; Susan J. Tolchin and Martin Tolchin, *Dismantling America: The Rush to Deregulate* (Boston: Houghton Mifflin, 1983), chap. 6, "Political Meltdown."

16. Phillip Knightley et al., *Suffer the Children: The Story of Thalidomide* (New York: Viking, 1979).

17. Richard Halloran, "Broad Criticism of Airline Safety Offered at Gander Crash Hearing," *The New York Times*, 6 February 1986, p. 9–B; Paul Eddy, Elaine Potter, and Bruce Page, *Destination Disaster—from the Tri–Motor to the DC–10: The Risks of Flying* (New York: Quadrangle, 1976).

18. Joan Claybrook and the Staff of Public Citizen, *Retreat from Safety: Reagan's Attack on America's Health* (New York: Pantheon, 1984); Tolchin and Tolchin, *Dismantling America*.

19. Kramer, p. 157.

20. Schrager and Short, p. 408; Francis T. Cullen, Bruce G. Link, and Craig W. Polanzi, "The Seriousness of Crime Revisited," *Criminology* 20 (May 1982), pp. 83–102; Francis T. Cullen et al., "Dissecting White-Collar Crime: Offense Type and Punitiveness," *International Journal of Comparative and Applied Criminal Justice* 9 (Spring 1985), pp. 15–28.

21. Mark Dowie, "The Corporate Crime of the Century," *Mother Jones* (November 1979), pp. 23–25 ff.; parts of this article are reprinted in this anthology under the title "The Dumping of Hazardous Products on Foreign Markets." See also Milton Silverman, Philip R. Lee, and Mia Lydecker, *Prescriptions for Death: The Drugging of the Third World* (Berkeley: University of California Press, 1982); John Braithwaite, *Corporate Crime in the Pharmaceutical Industry* (London: Routledge & Kegan Paul, 1984), chap. 7; Barry I. Castleman, "The Double Standard in Industrial Hazards," *Multinational Monitor* (September 1984), pp. 4–8.

22. Dowie, p. 24; Morton Mintz, *At Any Cost: Corporate Greed, Women, and the Dalkon Shield* (New York: Pantheon Books Inc., 1985).

23. Dowie, p. 24.

24. "Met-Ed Admits Falsifying TMI Records," *Syracuse Post-Dispatch*, 29 February 1984, p. 1; "Faking it at 3 Mile Island?" *The New York Times*, 12 November 1983, p. 8–E.

25. Mark Dowie, "Pinto Madness," *Mother Jones* (September-October 1977), pp. 18–32, reprinted in this anthology; Ronald C. Kramer, "Corporate Crime: An Organizational Perspective," in Peter Wickman and Timothy Daily, eds., *White-Collar and Economic Crime* (Lexington, Mass.: Lexington Books, 1982), pp. 75–94.

26. "GM X-Car Papers Said Brakes Had Problems," *Syracuse Post-Dispatch*, 21 October 1983, p. D–7; "GM Has More X-Car Problems," *The New York Times*, 26 August 1984, p. 2–E.

27. Kramer, "A Prolegomenon to the Study of Corporate Violence," p. 167.

28. Robert Jackall, "Crime in the Suites," *Contemporary Sociology* 9 (May 1980), p. 356.

29. Steven Box, *Power, Crime, and Mystification* (London: Tavistock, 1983), p. 21. See also Hannah Arendt, *Eichmann in Jerusalem: A Report on the Banality of Evil* (New York: Viking Press, 1963).

Part I

The Consumer as Victim

IN THE first article, "Pinto Madness," Mark Dowie reveals secret documents that show that the Ford Motor Company, for seven years, knowingly sold cars in which hundreds of people would needlessly burn to death. In 1978, the Department of Transportation finally pressured Ford to recall the Pinto subcompact after DOT tests conclusively documented the fuel-tank safety defects exposed in Dowie's article, which was first published in 1977. A grand jury in Elkhard, Indiana subsequently indicted the Ford Motor Company on charges of reckless homicide in connection with the death of three teenage women when the Pinto they were driving exploded and burned after being struck from behind. Although the prosecutor who brought unprecedented criminal charges against this powerful automobile manufacturer was unsuccessful in gaining a conviction, this landmark case represents a growing movement to hold corporations legally responsible for knowingly keeping on the market a life-threatening product and failing to inform the public of the hazards.

In the article "At Any Cost," medical writer Morton Mintz describes the immense suffering of thousands of women, at least eighteen of whom died, from using the defective Dalkon Shield intrauterine birth control device manufactured by the A.H. Robins Company. Mintz contends that despite growing evidence of the serious health hazards of this IUD, including pelvic infection, infertility, and birth defects, Robins officials used stonewalling tactics to deny such dangers and, for years, refused to warn the female users at risk.

At the settlement of a civil suit brought on behalf of seven women who were seriously harmed from using the Dalkon Shield, the presiding federal judge, Miles Lord, issued his own stinging reprimand (reprinted here under the title "A Plea for Corporate Conscience) to three top officials of the Robins company for their complicity in this avoidable tragedy.

In the final article in this section, "The Dumping of Hazardous Products on Foreign Markets," an investigative team under the direc-

11

tion of Mark Dowie, a contributing editor to *Mother Jones* magazine, documents the increasing dangers from exporting toxic pesticides, carcinogenic garments, unsafe drugs, and other dangerous products banned in the United States. The article describes some of the methods used to circumvent regulatory agencies in this country and suspicious importers abroad, as American corporations often fail to inform the users in foreign countries of the actual hazardous risks involved. Dowie outlines several measures to help protect consumers from this worldwide dumping of toxic substances and unsafe products by multinational corporations.

After growing publicity on corporate dumping overseas, President Jimmy Carter issued an executive order mandating stricter controls on the export of products banned in the United States. President Reagan revoked the order contending that such restrictions damage this country's balance of trade, encourage domestic manufacturers to shift their operations overseas, and decrease the sales of American-made goods with no benefits to Third World nations, who can import the same hazardous products from other industrial nations. The Reagan Administration instead encouraged American regulatory agencies who ban products from the domestic market to communicate more effectively with foreign ministries. As Dowie's article makes clear, however, the injurious consequences of dumping are not restricted only to poorly developed nations. In an ironic boomerang effect, government spot checks show that about ten percent of food imported to the United States—such as green coffee beans, melons, and bananas—is contaminated with illegal levels of potentially carcinogenic pesticides previously banned in this country.

1 / *Pinto Madness*

MARK DOWIE

ONE EVENING in the mid-1960s, Arjay Miller was driving home from his office in Dearborn, Michigan, in the four-door Lincoln Continental that went with his job as president of the Ford Motor Company. On a crowded highway, another car struck his from the rear. The Continental spun around and burst into flames. Because he was wearing a shoulder-strap seat belt, Miller was unharmed by the crash, and because his doors didn't jam he escaped the flaming wreck. But the accident made a vivid impression on him. Several months later, on July 15, 1965, he recounted it to a U.S. Senate subcommittee that was hearing testimony on auto safety legislation. "I still have burning in my mind the image of that gas tank on fire," Miller said. He went on to express an almost passionate interest in controlling fuel-fed fires in cars that crash or roll over. He spoke with excitement about the fabric gas tank Ford was testing at that very moment. "If it proves out," he promised the senators, "it will be a feature you will see in our standard cars."

Almost seven years after Miller's testimony, a woman, whom for legal reasons we will call Sandra Gillespie, pulled onto a Minneapolis highway in her new Ford Pinto. Riding with her was a young boy, whom we'll call Robbie Carlton. As she entered a merge lane, Sandra Gillespie's car stalled. Another car rear-ended hers at an impact speed of 28 miles per hour. The Pinto's gas tank ruptured. Vapors from it mixed quickly with the air in the passenger compartment. A spark ignited the mixture and the car exploded in a ball of fire. Sandra died in agony a few hours later in an emergency hospital. Her passenger, 13-year-old Robbie Carlton, is still alive; he has just come home from another futile operation aimed at grafting a new ear and nose from skin on the few unscarred portions of his badly burned body. (This accident is real; the details are from police reports.)

Why did Sandra Gillespie's Ford Pinto catch fire so easily, seven years after Ford's Arjay Miller made his apparently sincere pronouncements—the same seven years that brought more safety improvements to cars than any other period in automotive history? An extensive investigation by *Mother Jones* over the past six months has found these answers:

Fighting strong competition from Volkswagen for the lucrative smallcar market, the Ford Motor Company rushed the Pinto into production in much less than the usual time.

Ford engineers discovered in the pre-production crash tests that rear-end collisions would rupture the Pinto's fuel system extremely easily.

Because assembly-line machinery was already tooled when engineers found this defect, top Ford officials decided to manufacture the car anyway—exploding gas tank and all—*even though Ford owned the patent on a much safer gas tank.*

For more than eight years afterwards, Ford successfully lobbied, with extraordinary vigor and some blatant lies, against a key government safety standard that would have forced the company to change the Pinto's fire-prone gas tank.

By conservative estimates Pinto crashes have caused 500 burn deaths to people who would not have been seriously injured if the car had not burst into flames. Burning Pintos have become such an embarrassment to Ford that its advertising agency J. Walter Thompson, dropped a line from the end of a radio spot that read "Pinto leaves you with that warm feeling."

Ford knows the Pinto is a firetrap, yet it has paid out millions to settle damage suits out of court, and it is prepared to spend millions more lobbying against safety standards. With a half million cars rolling off the assembly line each year, Pinto is the biggest-selling subcompact in America, and the company's operating profit on the car is fantastic. Finally, in 1977, new Pinto models have incorporated a few minor alterations necessary to meet that federal standard Ford managed to hold off for eight years. Why did the company delay so long in making these minimal, inexpensive improvements?

Ford waited eight years because its internal "cost-benefit analysis," *which places a dollar value on human life,* said it wasn't profitable to make the changes sooner.

Before we get to the question of how much Ford thinks your life is worth, let's trace the history of the death trap itself. Although this particular story is about the Pinto, the way in which Ford made its decision is typical of the U.S. auto industry generally. There are plenty of similar stories about other cars made by other companies. But this case is the worst of them all.

The next time you drive behind a Pinto (with over two million of them on the road, you shouldn't have much trouble finding one), take a look at the rear end. That long silver object hanging down under the bumper is the gas tank. The tank begins about six inches forward of the bumper. In late models the bumper is designed to withstand a collision of only about five miles per hour. Earlier bumpers may as well not have been on the car for all the protection they offered the gas tank.

Mother Jones has studied hundreds of reports and documents on rear-end collisions involving Pintos. These reports conclusively reveal that if you ran into that Pinto you were following at over 30 miles per hour, the rear end of the car would buckle like an accordion, right up to the back seat. The tube leading to the gas-tank cap would be ripped away from the tank itself, and gas would immediately begin sloshing onto the road around the car. The buckled gas tank would be jammed up against the differential housing which contains four sharp protruding bolts likely to gash holes in the tank and spill still more gas. The welded seam between the main body frame and the wheel well would split, allowing gas to enter the interior of the car.

Now all you need is a spark from a cigarette, ignition, or scraping metal, and both cars would be engulfed in flames. If you gave the Pinto a really good whack—say, at 40 mph—chances are excellent that its doors would jam and you would have to stand by and watch its trapped passengers burn to death.

This scenario is no news to Ford. Internal company documents in our possession show that Ford has crash-tested the Pinto at a top-secret site more than 40 times and that *every* test made at over 25 mph without special structural alteration of the car has resulted in a ruptured fuel tank. Despite this, Ford officials denied having crash-tested the Pinto.

Eleven of these tests, averaging a 31-mph impact speed, came before Pintos started rolling out of the factories. Only three cars passed the test with unbroken fuel tanks. In one of them an inexpensive light-weight metal baffle was placed so those bolts would not perforate the tank. (Don't forget about that baffle which costs about a dollar and weighs about a pound. It plays an important role in our story later on.) In another successful test, a piece of steel was placed between the tank and the bumper. In the third test car the gas tank was lined with a rubber bladder. But none of these protective alterations was used in the mass-produced Pinto.

In preproduction planning, engineers seriously considered using in the Pinto the same kind of gas tank Ford uses in the Capri. The Capri tank rides over the rear axle and differential housing. It has been so successful in over 50 crash tests that Ford used it in its Experimental Safety Vehicle, which withstood rear-end impacts of 60 mph. So why wasn't the Capri tank used in the Pinto? Or, why wasn't that baffle placed between the tank and the axle—something that would have saved the life of Sandra Gillespie and hundreds like her. Why was a car known to be a serious fire hazard deliberately released to production in August of 1970?

Whether Ford should manufacture subcompacts at all was the subject of a bitter two-year debate at the company's Dearborn headquarters. The principals in this corporate struggle were the then-president Semon "Bunky" Knudsen, whom Henry Ford II had hired away from General Motors, and Lee Iacocca, a spunky young turk who had risen fast within the company on the enormous success of the Mustang. Iacocca argued forcefully that Volkswagen and the Japanese were going to capture the entire American subcompact market unless Ford put out its own alternative to the VW Beetle. Bunky Knudsen said, in effect: let them have the small-car market; Ford makes good money on medium and large models. But he lost the battle and later resigned. Iacocca became president and almost immediately began a rush program to produce the Pinto.

Like the Mustang, the Pinto became known in the company as "Lee's car." Lee Iacocca wanted that little car in the showrooms of America with the 1971 models. So he ordered his engineering vice president, Bob Alexander, to oversee what was probably the shortest production planning period in modern automotive history. The normal time span from conception to production of a new car model is about 43 months. The Pinto Schedule was set at just under 25.

Design, styling, product planning, advance engineering and quality assurance all have flexible time frames, and engineers can pretty much carry these on simultaneously. Tooling, on the other hand, has a fixed time frame of about 18 months. Normally, an auto company doesn't begin tooling until the other processes are almost over. *But Iacocca's speed-up meant Pinto tooling went on at the same time as product development.* So when crash tests revealed a serious defect in the gas tank, it was too late. The tooling was well under way.

When it was discovered the gas tank was unsafe, did anyone go to Iacocca and tell him? "Hell no," replied an engineer who worked on the Pinto, a high company official for many years, who, unlike several others at Ford, maintains a necessarily clandestine concern for safety. "That person would have been fired. Safety wasn't a popular subject around Ford in those days. With Lee it was taboo. Whenever a problem was raised that meant a delay on the Pinto, Lee would chomp on his cigar, look out the window and say 'Read the product objectives and get back to work."

The product objectives are clearly stated in the Pinto "green book." This is a thick, top-secret manual in green covers containing a step-by-step production plan for the model, detailing the metallurgy, weight, strength and quality of every part in the car. The product objectives for the Pinto are repeated in an article by Ford executive F. G. Olsen published by the Society of Automotive Engineers. He lists these product objectives as follows:

1. TRUE SUBCOMPACT
   • Size
   • Weight
2. LOW COST OF OWNERSHIP
   • Initial price
   • Fuel consumption
   • Reliability
   • Serviceability
3. CLEAR PRODUCT SUPERIORITY
   • Appearance
   • Comfort
   • Features
   • Ride and Handling
   • Performance

Safety, you will notice, is not there. It is not mentioned in the entire article. As Lee Iacocca was fond of saying, "Safety doesn't sell."

Heightening the anti-safety pressure on Pinto engineers was an important goal set by Iacocca known as "the limits of 2,000." The Pinto was not to weight an ounce over 2,000 pounds and not to cost a cent over $2,000. "Iacocca enforced these limits with an iron hand," recalls the engineer quoted earlier. So, even when a crash test showed that that one-pound, one-dollar piece of metal stopped the puncture of the gas tank, it was thrown out as extra cost and extra weight.

People shopping for subcompacts are watching every dollar. "You have to keep in mind," the engineer explained, "that the price elasticity on these subcompacts is extremely tight. You can price yourself right out of the market by adding $25 to the production cost of the model. And nobody understands that better than Iacocca."

Dr. Leslie Ball, the retired safety chief for the NASA manned space program and a founder of the International Society of Reliability Engineers, recently made a careful study of the Pinto. "The release to production of the Pinto was the most reprehensible decision in the history of American engineering," he said. Ball can name more than 40 European and Japanese models in the Pinto price and weight range with safer gas-tank positioning. Ironically, many of them, like the Ford Capri, contain a "saddle-style" gas tank riding over the back axle. *The patent on the saddle-type tank is owned by the Ford Motor Co.*

Los Angeles auto safety expert Byron Bloch has made an in-depth study of the Pinto fuel system. "It's a catastrophic blunder," he says.

"Ford made an extremely irresponsible decision when they placed such a weak tank in such a ridiculous location in such a soft rear end. It's almost designed to blow up—premeditated."

A Ford engineer, who doesn't want his name used, comments: "This company is run by salesmen, not engineers: so the priority is styling, not safety." He goes on to tell a story about gas-tank safety at Ford:

Lou Tubben is one of the most popular engineers at Ford. He's a friendly, outgoing guy with a genuine concern for safety. By 1971 he had grown so concerned about gas-tank integrity that he asked his boss if he could prepare a presentation on safer tank design. Tubben and his boss had both worked on the Pinto and shared a concern for its safety. His boss gave him the go-ahead, scheduled a date for the presentation and invited all company engineers and key production planning personnel. When time came for the meeting, a total of two people showed up—Lou Tubben and his boss.

"So you see," continued the anonymous Ford engineer, "there *are* a few of us here at Ford who are concerned about fire safety." He adds: "They are mostly engineers who have to study a lot of accident reports and look at pictures of burned people. But we don't talk about it much. It isn't a popular subject. I've never seen safety on the agenda of a product meeting and, except for a brief period in 1956, can't remember seeing the word safety in an advertisement. I really don't think the company wants American consumers to start thinking too much about safety—for fear they might demand it, I suppose."

Asked about the Pinto gas tank, another Ford engineer admitted: "That's all true. But you miss the point entirely. You see, safety isn't the issue, trunk space is. You have no idea how stiff the competition is over trunk space. Do you realize that if we put a Capri-type tank in the Pinto you could only get one set of golf clubs in the trunk?"

Blame for Sandra Gillespie's death, Robbie Carlton's unrecognizable face and all the other injuries and deaths in Pinto's since 1970 does not rest on the shoulders of Lee Iacocca alone. For, while he and his associates fought their battle against a safer Pinto in Dearborn, a larger war against safer cars raged in Washington. One skirmish in that war involved Ford's successful eight-year lobbying effort against Federal Motor Vehicle Safety Standard 301, the rear-end provisions of which would have forced Ford to redesign the Pinto.

But first some background:

During the early '60s, auto safety legislation became the *bête-noire* of American big business. The auto industry was the last great unregulated business, and if *it* couldn't reverse the tide of government regulation, the reasoning went, no one could.

People who know him cannot remember Henry Ford taking a

stronger stand than the one he took against the regulation of safety design. He spent weeks in Washington calling on members of Congress, holding press conferences and recruiting business cronies like W. B. Murphy of Campbell's Soup to join the anti-regulation battle. Displaying the sophistication for which today's American corporate leaders will be remembered, Murphy publicly called auto safety "a hula hoop, a fad that will pass." He was speaking to a special luncheon of the Business Council, an organization of 100 chief executives who gather periodically in Washington to provide "advice" and "counsel" to government. The target of their wrath in this instance was the Motor Vehicle Safety Bills introduced in both houses of Congress, largely in response to Ralph Nader's *Unsafe at Any Speed.*

By 1965, most pundits and lobbyists saw the handwriting on the wall and prepared to accept government "meddling" in the last bastion of free enterprise. Not Henry. With bulldog tenacity, he held out for defeat of the legislation to the very end, loyal to his grandfather's invention and to the company that makes it. But the Safety Act passed the House and Senate unanimously, and was signed into law by Lyndon Johnson in 1966.

While lobbying for and against legislation is pretty much a process of high-level back-slapping, press-conferencing and speech-making, fighting a regulatory agency is a much subtler matter. Henry headed home to lick his wounds in Grosse Pointe, Michigan, and a planeload of the Ford Motor Company's best brains flew to Washington to start the "education" of the new federal auto safety bureaucrats.

Their job was to implant the official industry ideology in the minds of the new officials regulating auto safety. Briefly summarized, that ideology states that auto accidents are caused not by *cars,* but by people and highway conditions.

It is an experience to hear automotive "safety engineers" talk for hours without ever mentioning cars. They will advocate spending billions educating youngsters, punishing drunks and redesigning street signs. Listening to them, you begin to think that it is easier to control 100 million drivers than a handful of manfacturers. They show movies about guardrail design and advocate the clear-cutting of trees 100 feet back from every highway in the nation. If a car is unsafe, they argue, it is because its owner doesn't maintain it properly.

In light of an annual death rate approaching 50,000, they are forced to admit that driving is hazardous. But the car is, in the words of Arjay Miller, "the safest link in the safety chain."

Before the Ford experts left Washington to return to drafting tables in Dearborn they did one other thing. They managed to informally reach an agreement with the major public servants who would be making auto safety decisions. This agreement was that "cost-benefit" would be an acceptable mode of analysis by Detroit and its new regulators. And, as we shall see, cost-benefit analysis quickly became the basis of Ford's argument against safer car design.

Cost-benefit analysis was used only occasionally in government until President Kennedy appointed Ford Motor Company President Robert McNamara to be Secretary of Defense. McNamara, originally an accountant, preached cost benefit with all the force of a Biblical zealot. Stated in its simplest terms, cost-benefit analysis says that if the cost is greater than the benefit, the project is not worth it—no matter what the benefit. Examine the cost of every action, decision, contract, part, or change, the doctrine says, then carefully evaluate the benefits (in dollars) to be certain that they exceed the cost before you begin a program or pass a regulation.

As a management tool in a business in which profits count over all else, cost-benefit analysis makes a certain amount of sense. Serious problems arise, however, when public officials who ought to have more than corporate profits at heart apply cost-benefit analysis to every conceivable decision. The inevitable result is that they must place a dollar value on human life.

Ever wonder what your life is worth in dollars? Perhaps $10 million? Ford has a better idea: $200,000.

Remember, Ford had gotten the federal regulators to agree to talk auto safety in terms of cost-benefit. But in order to be able to argue that various safety costs were greater than their benefits, Ford needed to have a dollar value figure for the "benefit." Rather than coming up with a price tag itself, the auto industry pressured the National Highway Traffic Safety Administration to do so. And in a 1972 report the agency determined that a human life lost on the highway was worth $200,725. Inflationary forces have recently pushed the figure up to $278,000.

Furnished with this useful tool, Ford immediately went to work using it to prove why various safety improvements were too expensive to make.

Nowhere did the company argue harder that it should make no changes than in the area of rupture-prone fuel tanks. Not long after the government arrived at the $200,725-per life figure, it surfaced, rounded off to a cleaner $200,000, in an internal Ford memorandum. This cost-benefit analysis argued that Ford should not make an $11-per-car improvement that would prevent 180 fiery deaths a year.

This cold calculus [Table 1] is buried in a seven-page company memorandum entitled "Fatalities Associated with Crash-Induced Fuel Leakage and Fires."

The memo goes on to argue that there is no financial benefit in complying with proposed safety standards that would admittedly

*Table 1   Benefits and Costs Relating to Fuel Leakage Associated with the Static
Rollover Test Portion of FMVSS 208*

Benefits

Savings: 180 burn deaths, 180 serious burn injuries, 2,100 burned vehicles.
Unit cost: $200,000 per death, $67,000 per injury, $700 per vehicle.
Total benefit: 180 × ($200,000) + 180 × ($67,000) + 2,100 × ($700) = $49.5 million.

Costs

Sales: 11 million cars, 1.5 million light trucks.
Unit cost: $11 per car, $11 per truck.
Total cost: 11,000,000 × ($11) + 1,500,000 × ($11) = $137 million.

result in fewer auto fires, fewer burn deaths and fewer burn injuries. Naturally, memoranda that speak so casually of "burn deaths" and "burn injuries" are not released to the public. They are very effective, however, with Department of Transportation officials indoctrinated in McNamarian cost-benefit analysis.

All Ford had to do was convince men like John Volpe, Claude Brinegar and William Coleman (successive Secretaries of Transportation during the Nixon-Ford years) that certain safety standards would add so much to the price of cars that fewer people would buy them. This could damage the auto industry, which was still believed to be the bulwark of the American economy. "Compliance to these standards," Henry Ford II prophesied at more than one press conference, "will shut down the industry."

The Nixon Transportation Secretaries were the kind of regulatory officials big business dreams of. They understood and loved capitalism and thought like businessmen. Yet, best of all, they came into office uninformed on technical automotive matters. And you could talk "burn injuries" and "burn deaths" with those guys, and they didn't seem to envision children crying at funerals and people hiding in their homes with melted faces. Their minds appeared to have leapt right to the bottom line—more safety meant higher prices, higher prices meant lower sales and lower sales meant lower profits.

So when J. C. Echold, Director of Automotive Safety (chief anti-safety lobbyist) for Ford wrote to the Department of Transportation—which he still does frequently, at great length—he felt secure attaching a memorandum that in effect says it is acceptable to kill 180 people and burn another 180 every year, *even though we have the technology that could save their lives for $11 a car.*

Furthermore, Echold attached this memo, confident, evidently, that the Secretary would question neither his low death/injury statistics nor his high cost estimates. But it turns out, on closer examination, that both these findings were midleading.

First, note that Ford's table shows an equal number of burn deaths and burn injuries. This is false. All independent experts estimate that for each person who dies by an auto fire, many more are left with charred hands, faces and limbs. Andrew McGuire of the Northern California Burn Center estimates the ratio of burn injuries to deaths at ten to one instead of the one to one Ford shows here. Even though Ford values a burn at only a piddling $67,000 instead of the $200,000 price of life, the true ratio obviously throws the company's calculations way off.

The other side of the equation, the alleged $11 cost of a fire-prevention device, is also a misleading estimation. One document that was *not* sent to Washington by Ford was a "Confidential" cost analysis *Mother Jones* has managed to obtain, showing that crash fires could be largely prevented for considerably *less* than $11 a car. The cheapest method involves placing a heavy rubber bladder inside the gas tank to keep the fuel from spilling if the tank ruptures. Goodyear had developed the bladder and had demonstrated it to the automotive industry. We have in our possession crash-test reports showing that the Goodyear bladder worked well. On December 2, 1970 (*two years before* Echold sent his cost-benefit memo to Washington), Ford Motor Company ran a rear-end crash test on a car with the rubber bladder in the gas tank. The tank ruptured, but no fuel leaked. On January 15, 1971, Ford again tested the bladder and again it worked. The total purchase and installation cost of the bladder would have been $5.08 per car. That $5.08 could have saved the lives of Sandra Gillespie and several hundred others.

When a federal regulatory agency like the National Highway Traffic Safety Administration (NHTSA) decides to issue a new standard, the law usually requires it to invite all interested parties to respond before the standard is enforced—a reasonable enough custom on the surface. However, the auto industry has taken advantage of this process and has used it to delay lifesaving emission and safety standards for years. In the case of the standard that would have corrected that fragile Pinto fuel tank, the delay was for an incredible eight years.

The particular regulation involved here was Federal Motor Vehicle Safety Standard 301. Ford picked portions of Standard 301 for strong opposition back in 1968 when the Pinto was still in the blueprint stage. The intent of 301, and the 300 series that followed it, was to protect drivers and passengers *after* a crash occurs. Without question the worst postcrash hazard is fire. So Standard 301 originally proposed that all cars should be able to withstand a fixed barrier impact of 20 mph (that is, running into a wall at that speed) without losing fuel.

When the standard was proposed, Ford engineers pulled their crash-test results out of their files. The front ends of most cars were no problem—with minor alterations they could stand the impact without losing fuel. "We were already working on the front end," Ford engineer Dick Kimble admitted. "We knew we could meet the test on the front end." But with the Pinto particularly, a 20-mph rear-end standard meant redesigning the entire rear end of the car. With the Pinto scheduled for production in August of 1970, and with $200 million worth of tools in place, adoption of this standard would have created a minor financial disaster. So Standard 301 was targeted for delay, and, with some assistance from its industry associates, Ford succeeded beyond its wildest expectations: the standard was not adopted until the 1977 model year. Here is how it happened:

There are several main techniques in the art of combating a government safety standard: a) make your arguments in succession, so the feds can be working on disproving only one at a time; b) claim that the real problem is not X but Y (we already saw one instance of this in "the problem is not cars but people"); c) no matter how ridiculous each argument is, accompany it with thousands of pages of highly technical assertions it will take the government months or, preferably, years to test. Ford's large and active Washington office brought these techniques to new heights and became the envy of the lobbyists' trade.

The Ford people started arguing against Standard 301 way back in 1968 with a strong attack of technique b). Fire, they said, was not the real problem. Sure, cars catch fire and people burn occasionally. But statistically auto fires are such a minor problem that NHTSA should really concern itself with other matters.

Strange as it may seem, the Department of Transportation (NHTSA's parent agency) didn't know whether or not this was true. So it contracted with several independent research groups to study auto fires. The studies took months, often years, which was just what Ford wanted. The completed studies, howevery, showed auto fires to be more of a problem than Transportation officials ever dreamed of. A Washington research firm found that 400,000 cars were burning up every year, burning more than 3,000 people to death. Furthermore, auto fires were increasing five times as fast as building fires. Another study showed that 35 per cent of all fire deaths in the U.S. occurred in automobiles. Forty per cent of all fire department calls in the 1960s were to vehicle fires—a public cost of $350 million a year, a figure that, incidentally, never shows up in cost-benefit analyses.

Another study was done by the Highway Traffic Research Institute in Ann Arbor, Michigan, a safety think-tank funded primarily by the auto industry (the giveaway there is the words "highway traffic" rather than "automobile" in the group's name). It concluded that 40 per cent of the lives lost in fuel-fed fires could be saved if the manufacturers complied with proposed Standard 301. Finally, a third report was prepared for NHTSA. This report indicated that the Ford Motor Company makes 24 per cent of the cars on the American road, yet these cars account for 42 per cent of the collison-ruptured fuel tanks.

Ford lobbyist then used technique a)—bringing up a new argument. Their line then became: yes, perhaps burn accidents do happen, but rear-end collisions are relatively rare (note the echo of technique b) here as well). Thus Standard 301 was not needed. This set the NHTSA off on a new round of analyzing accident reports. The government's findings finally were that rear-end collisions were seven and a half times more likely to result in fuel spills than were front-end collisions. So much for that argument.

By now it was 1972; NHTSA had been researching and analyzing for four years to answer Ford's objections. During that time, nearly 9,000 people burned to death in flaming wrecks. Tens of thousands more were badly burned and scarred for life. And the four-year delay meant that well over 10 million new unsafe vehicles went on the road, vehicles that will be crashing, leaking fuel and incinerating people well into the 1980s.

Ford now had to enter its third round of battling the new regulations. On the "the problem is not X but Y" principle, the company had to look around for something new to get itself off the hook. One might have thought that, faced with all the latest statistics on the horrifying number of deaths in flaming accidents, Ford would find the task difficult. But the company's rhetoric was brilliant. The problem was not burns, but . . . impact! Most of the people killed in these fiery accidents, claimed Ford, would have died whether the car burned or not. They were killed by the kinetic force of the impact, not the fire.

And so once again, the ball bounced into the government's court and the absurdly pro-industry NHTSA began another slow-motion response. Once again it began a time-consuming round of test crashes and embarked on a study of accidents. The latter, however, revealed that a large and growing number of corpses taken from burned cars involved in rear-end crashes contained no cuts, bruises or broken bones. They clearly would have survived the accident unharmed if the cars had not caught fire. This pattern was confirmed in careful rear-end crash tests performed by the Insurance Institute for Highway Safety. A University of Miami study found an inordinate number of Pintos burning on rear-end impact and concluded that this demonstrated "a clear and present hazard to all Pinto owners."

Pressure on NHTSA from Ralph Nader and consumer groups began mounting. The industry-agency collusion was so obvious that Senator Joseph Montoya (D-N.M.) introduced legislation about Standard 301. NHTSA waffled some more and again announced its intentions to promulgate a rear-end collision standard.

Waiting, as it normally does, until the last day allowed for response, Ford filed with NHTSA a gargantuan batch of letters, studies and charts now arguing that the federal testing criteria were unfair. Ford also argued that design changes required to meet the standard would take 43 months which seemed like a rather long time in light of the fact that the entire Pinto was designed in about two years. Specifically new complaints about the standard involved the weight of the test vehicle, whether or not the brakes should be engaged at the moment of impact and the claim that the standard should only apply to cars, not trucks or buses. Perhaps the most amusing argument was that the engine should not be idling during crash tests, the rationale being that an idling engine meant that the gas tank had to contain gasoline and that the hot lights needed to film the crash might ignite the gasoline and cause a fire.

Some of these complaints were accepted, others rejected. But they all required examination and testing by a week kneed NHTSA, meaning more of those 18-month studies the industry loves so much. So the complaints served their real purpose—delay; all told, an eight-year delay, while Ford manufactured more than three million profitable, dangerously incendiary Pintos. To justify his delay, Henry Ford II called more press conferences to predict the demise of American civlization. "If we can't meet the standards when they are published," he warned, "we will have to close down. And if we have to close down some production because we don't meet standards we're in for real trouble in this country."

While government bureaucrats dragged their feet on lifesaving Standard 301, a different kind of expert was taking a close look at the Pinto—the "recon man." "Recon" stands for reconstruction; recon men reconstruct accidents for police departments, insurance companies and lawyers who want to know exactly who or what caused an accident. It didn't take many rear-end Pinto accidents to demonstrate the weakness of the car. Recon men began encouraging lawyers to look beyond one driver or another to the manufacturer in their search for fault, particularly in the growing number of accidents where passengers were uninjured by collision but were badly burned by fire.

Pinto lawsuits began mounting fast against Ford. Says John Versace, executive safety engineer at Ford's Safety Research Center, "Ulcers are running pretty high among the engineers who worked on the Pinto. Every lawyer in the country seems to want to take their depositions." (The Safety Research Center is an impressive glass and concrete building standing by itself about a mile from Ford World Headquarters in Dearborn. Looking at it, one imagines its large staff protects consumers from burned and broken limbs. Not so. The Center is the technical support arm of Jack Echold's 14-person anti-regulatory lobbying team in World Headquarters.)

When the Pinto liability suits began, Ford strategy was to go to a jury. Confident it could hide the Pinto crash tests, Ford thought that juries of solid American registered voters would buy the industry doctrine that drivers, not cars, cause accidents. It didn't work. It seems that citizens are much quicker to see the truth than bureaucracies. Juries began ruling against the company, granting million-dollar awards to plaintiffs.

"We'll never go to a jury again," says Al Slechter in Ford's Washington office. "Not in a fire case. Juries are just too sentimental. They see those charred remains and forget the evidence. No sir, we'll settle."

Settlement involves less cash, smaller legal fees and less publicity, but it is an indication of the weakness of their case. Nevertheless, Ford has been offering to settle when it is clear that the company can't pin the blame on the driver of the other car. But, since the company carries $2 million deductible product-liability insurance these settlements have a direct impact on the bottom line. They must therefore be considered a factor in determining the net operating profit on the Pinto. It's impossible to get a straight answer from Ford on the profitability of the Pinto and the impact of lawsuit settlements on it— even when you have a curious and mildly irate shareholder call to inquire, as we did. However, financial officer Charles Matthews did admit that the company establishes a reserve for large dollar settlements. He would not divulge the amount of the reserve and had no explanation for its absence from the annual report.

Until recently, it was clear that, whatever the cost of these settlements, it was not enough to seriously cut into the Pinto's enormous profits. The cost of retooling Pinto assembly lines and of equipping each car with a safety gadget like that $5.08 Goodyear bladder was, company accountants calculated, greater than that of paying out millions to survivors like Robbie Carlton or to widows and widowers of victims like Sandra Gillespie. The bottom line ruled, and inflammable Pintos kept rolling out of the factories.

In 1977, however, an incredibly sluggish government has at last instituted Standard 301. New Pintos will have to have rupture-proof gas tanks. Or will they?

To everyone's surprise, the 1977 Pinto recently passed a rear-end crash test in Phoenix, Arizona, for NHTSA. The agency was so convinced the Pinto would fail that it was the first car tested. Amazingly, it did not burst into flame.

"We have had so many Ford failures in the past," explained agency engineer Tom Grubbs, "I felt sure the Pinto would fail."

How did it pass?

Remember that one-dollar, one-pound metal baffle that was on one of the three modified Pintos that passed the pre-production crash tests nearly ten years ago? Well, it is a standard feature on the 1977 Pinto. In the Phoenix test it protected the gas tank from being perforated by those four bolts on the differential housing.

We asked Grubbs if he noticed any other substantial alterations in the rear-end structure of the car. "No," he replied, "the [baffle] seems to be the only noticeable change over the 1976 model."

But was it? What Tom Grubbs and the Department of Transportation didn't know when they tested the car was that it was manufactured in St. Thomas, Ontario. Ontario? The significance of that becomes clear when you learn that Canada has for years had extremely strict rear-end collision standards.

Tom Irwin is the business manager of Charlie Rossi Ford, the Scottsdale, Arizona, dealership that sold the Pinto to Tom Grubbs. He refused to explain why he was selling Fords made in Canada when there is a huge Pinto assembly plant much closer by in California. "I know why you're asking that question, and I'm not going to answer it," he blurted out. "You'll have to ask the company."

But Ford's regional office in Phoenix has "no explanation" for the presence of Canadian cars in their local dealership. Farther up the line in Dearborn, Ford people claim there is absolutely no difference between American and Canadian Pintos. They say cars are shipped back and forth across the border as a matter of course. But they were hard pressed to explain why some Canadian Pintos were shipped all the way to Scottsdale, Arizona. Significantly, one engineer at the St. Thomas plant did admit that the existence of strict rear-end collision standards in Canada "might encourage us to pay a little more attention to quality control on that part of the car."

The Department of Transportation is considering buying an American Pinto and running the test again. For now, it will only say that the situation is under investigation.

Whether the new American Pinto fails or passes the test, Standard 301 will never force the company to test or recall the more than two million pre-1977 Pintos still on the highway. Seventy or more people will burn to death in those cars every year for many years to come. If the past is any indication, Ford will continue to accept the deaths.

According to safety expert Byron Bloch, the older cars could quite easily be retrofitted with gas tanks containing fuel cells. "These improved tanks would add at least 10 mph improved safety performance to the rear end," he estimated, "but it would cost Ford $20 to $30 a car, so they won't do it unless they are forced to." Dr. Kenneth Saczalski, safety engineer with the Office of Naval Research in Washington, agrees. "The Defense Department has developed virtually fail-safe fuel systems and retrofitted them into existing vehicles. We have shown them to the auto industry and they have ignored them."

Unfortunately, the Pinto is not an isolated case of corporate malpractice in the auto industry. Neither is Ford a lone sinner. There probably isn't a car on the road without a safety hazard known to its manufacturer. And though Ford may have the best auto lobbyists in Washington, it is not alone. The anti-emission control lobby and the anti-safety lobby usually work in chorus form, presenting a well-harmonized message from the country's richest industry, spoken through the voices of individual companies—the Motor Vehicle Manufacturers Association, the Business Council and the U.S. Chamber of Commerce.

Furthermore, cost-valuing human life is not used by Ford alone.

Table 2   *What's Your Life Worth? Societal Cost Components for Fatalities, 1972 NHTSA Study*

Component	1971 Costs
Future productivity losses	
Direct	$132,000
Indirect	41,300
Medical costs	
Hospital	700
Other	425
Property damage	1,500
Insurance administration	4,700
Legal and court	3,000
Employer losses	1,000
Victim's pain and suffering	10,000
Funeral	900
Assets (lost consumption)	5,000
Miscellaneous accident cost	200
Total per fatality: $200,725	

Here is a chart from a federal study showing how the National Highway Traffic Safety Administration has calculated the value of a human life. The estimate was arrived at under pressure from the auto industry. The Ford Motor Company has used it in cost-benefit analyses arguing why certain safety measures are not "worth" the savings in human lives. The calculation above is a breakdown of the estimated cost to society every time someone is killed in a car accident. We were not able to find anyone, either in the government or at Ford, who could explain how the $10,000 figure for "pain and suffering" had been arrived at.

Ford was just the only company careless enough to let such an embarrassing calculation slip into public records. The process of willfully trading lives for profits goes back at least as far as Commodore Vanderbilt, who publicly scorned George Westinghouse and his "foolish" air brakes while people died by the hundreds in accidents on Vanderbilt's railroads.

The original draft of the Motor Vehicle Safety Act provided for criminal sanction against a manufacturer who willfully placed an unsafe car on the market. Early in the proceedings the auto industry lobbied the provision out of the bill. Since then, there have been those damage settlements, of course, but the only government punishment meted out to auto companies for non-compliance to standards has been a minuscule fine, usually $5,000 to $10,000. One wonders how long the Ford Motor Company would continue to market lethal cars were Henry Ford II and Lee Iacocca serving 20-year terms in Leavenworth for consumer homicide.

2 / At Any Cost: Corporate Greed, Women, and the Dalkon Shield

MORTON MINTZ

In January 1971, the A.H. Robins company began to sell the Dalkon Shield, promoting it as the "modern, superior," "second generation," and, most important, "safe" intrauterine device for birth control. Robins, a major pharmaceutical manufacturer in Richmond, Virginia, distributed 4.5 million of the IUDs in eighty countries before halting sales in the mid-1970s. There followed a catastrophe without precedent in the annals of medicine and law.

The story of the Dalkon Shield lays bare the perils inherent in contemporary business practices and in corporate law, in a system that allows corporations to profit even if they put human beings at risk. The Shield created a disaster of global proportions because a few men with little on their minds except the pursuit of megabucks made decisions, in the interest of profit, that exposed millions of women to serious infection, sterility, and even death. To be sure, the same pursuit finally led Robins, in August 1985, to seek reorganization under Chapter 11 of the Bankruptcy Code. For the uncompensated victims, this may be yet another blow because, critics fear, reorganization could let the company put them at the end of a line of lenders, suppliers, and other creditors.

The problem at the core of such conduct is not simply that corporations have no conscience, but that they are endowed by law with rights beyond those allowed to individuals. Corporations too often act without compassion and, no matter what damage they cause, without remorse. Even worse, they cannot be held accountable, as people can be. You cannot lock up a corporation, or sentence it to hard labor or to the electric chair. And too often the law fails to look behind the corporate veil, to prosecute the individuals who make decisions and act in the name of the corporation.

30

[A human being who would not harm you on an individual face-to-face basis, who is charitable, civic-minded, loving, and devout, will wound or kill you from behind the corporate veil. He may do this without qualm because he has been conditioned to drop a curtain betweeen his private moral and religious self and his corporate immoral and irreligious self. Society at large accepts and, if only by its silence, *validates* such compartmentalization.]

Worldwide, the seriously injured victims of the Dalkon Shield could number in the tens of thousands. Nearly all suffered life-threatening forms of the infections known as pelvic inflammatory disease (PID). In the United States alone, PID killed at least eighteen women who had been wearing Shields. Most of the infections impaired or destroyed the women's ability to bear children.

Not only was the Shield unsafe, it was surprisingly ineffective. The number of wearers who became pregnant with the devices in place was on the order of 110,000, or 5 per cent, a rate nearly five times the one falsely claimed in advertising and promotion to physicians and women, and a rate sharply higher than that for many other IUDs. The exaggerated and bogus claim led women to reject more effective birth control in favor of the Shield, and this led directly to consequences far worse than unwanted pregnancies.

An estimated 60 per cent of the U.S. women who conceived with Shields in place lost their unborn, or about 10,000 more than would have done so had they been wearing other IUDs. Some of these women had elective abortions. Others suffered the previously rare miscarriages called *spontaneous abortions*. Others, in the fourth to sixth months of pregnancy, experienced the still rarer infected miscarriages, or *septic spontaneous abortions*. By the count of the Food and Drug Administration (FDA), 248 women, just in this country, endured this dangerous, Shield-related complication. For fifteen of them, these septic abortions were fatal.

Hundreds of women throughout the world who conceived while wearing the Shield gave birth prematurely, in the final trimester, to children with grave congenital defects, including blindness, cerebral palsy, and mental retardation. No one can pinpoint the exact number of such women, partly because no one knows how many times women or their doctors failed to make a proper connection between the Shield and the premature birth of a defective baby.

Robins distributed about 2.86 million Shields in the United States, and doctors implanted them, by the company's estimate, in 2.2 million women. Abroad, Robins distributed about 1.71 million Shields, and in June 1974 it estimated that 800,000 to one million were implanted.

In 1974, increasing and alarming numbers of Shield-related spontaneous septic abortions became known to the FDA, and the agency asked Robins to suspend Shield sales in the United States. It did so on June 28, 1974.

In 1975, a year after the suspension of Shield salaes here, Martina Langley was a volunteer at a family-planning clinic in El Salvador. Now a lawyer in Austin, Texas, she recalls that the only IUD the clinic's doctors were inserting was the Shield, and that some clinics in El Salvador continued to implant Shields until 1980.

"Sometimes the doctor would say to the patient, 'This is from the United States and it's very good,'" Langley told David Phelps, a Washington correspondent for the *Minneapolis Star and Tribune*. Then, she said, the doctor would motion toward her and tell the woman, "She is from the United States and people [there] use it." Figures are simply unavailable from most of the countries where the Shield was used. My guess is that Shield-related PID killed hundreds—possibly thousands—of women outside of the United States.

Dr. Richard P. Dickey, a former member of the Food and Drug Administration's obstetrical and gynecological devices advisory panel, has seen first-hand the conditions faced by a woman who suffers PID. An infected Shield wearer "where there are no doctors, no antibiotics, she's going to die," he told me.

Today, more than a decade after Shield sales officially ended in the United States, its legacies of death, disease, injury, and pain persist. Even women who have had the Shield removed are not out of danger. Because PID is commonly not an affliction that is simply treated and is then over and done with, large numbers of Dalkon Shield wearers suffer chronic pain and illness, sometimes requiring repeated hospitalization and surgery. Many have waged desperate battles to bear children despite severe damage to their reproductive systems.

More cheerless news came last April from two studies funded by the National Institutes of Health. They showed that childless IUD wearers who have had PID run a far higher risk of infertility if their devices were Shields than if they were other makes. Not even women who still wear the Shield with no apparent problem are safe: They run the risk of suddenly being stricken by life-threatening PID. In the words of Miles W. Lord, who retired recently as Chief District Judge for Minnesota, they are wearing "a deadly depth charge in their wombs, ready to explode at any time."

The exact number of women still wearing the Shield is unknown. By early 1983, some FDA officials and gynecologists were confident that few American women, probably only hundreds, still used it. Other qualified observers, however, were estimating the figure to be much higher, anywhere from 80,000 to more than half a million.

Certainly the response to Robins's own call-back campaign of October 1984 suggests the higher figures are closer to the mark. By

February 1, 1985, a $4 million advertising drive, which urged women still wearing the Shields to have them removed at Robins's expense, had drawn more than 16,000 telephone calls on toll-free hotlines; by the end of March, 4,437 women had filed claims for Shield removals. The claims were flowing in at the dramatic rate of more than 100 a week.

Mary Beth Kornhauser, screenwriter in West Hollywood, California, was thirty-one when I interviewed her last December. In its essentials, her story is similar to that of countless other women whose quest for safe and effective birth control led them to trust their physicians, who in turn trusted the manufacturer.

Mary was first fitted with a Shield when she was eighteen. She began having dangerous, extremely painful, and recurring pelvic infections. From the start, her misfortune was compounded by physicians whose incompetent diagnoses, such as that she was experiencing a nervous breakdown, destroyed her chances for a full and swift recovery.

In October 1972, one physician pronounced her seriously infected and removed her Shield; he did not properly treat the infection and intimated that she had gotten it because of a promiscuous life style. After seven terrible years of misdiagnosis and illness she was finally deprived of her ability to bear a child. Here is her description of the events directly preceding the "total hysterectomy" she suffered at age twenty-five:

"In 1978, I started getting sick cramps, vomiting, high fever, the same spells that had come up periodically. I went to a doctor, and he gave me oral antibiotics, which didn't work. So I went back to the University of California at Los Angeles Medical Center, where a doctor recommended me to . . . Dr. Charles E. Hamrell in Santa Monica, and he immediately put me in the hospital.

"I was very infected with tubo-ovarian abscesses, one the size of a grapefruit, one the size of an orange. I was apparently about ready to explode. To try to control the infection to prevent it from spilling into the abdominal cavity, Dr. Hamrell put me in Santa Monica Hospital for serious intravenous antibiotic therapy, by which I mean that three different antibiotics were pumped into me, one each hour."

After eight days in the hospital, Mary returned to her apartment, sensing that she was only having a reprieve: Hamrell had prepared her for the possibility of a radical hysterectomy. She took antibiotics orally and was cared for by her sister, who flew in from the Midwest, and her mother, who came from Maryland. Two weeks later, Hamrell had to operate. It was February 15, 1979—one day less than seven years after her Dalkon Shield had been inserted.

Mary filed suit against Robins in November 1979. When her lawyer,

John T. Baker, prepared a "statement of facts," she said, "it read like Watergate, except that this was my life. You know, charges such as reckless disregard of truth, fraud. The reality of seeing this in print, it was staggering. But the real truth was that what they did was criminal, and that criminal charges should have been brought against the persons responsible.

"That there was a conspiracy by Robins executives to hide the truth is what got me. The fact that Americans, especially in pharmaceutical companies, would so knowingly ravage women, and get away with it, was staggering. . . . You'd think that when people deal in pharmaceutical medicine, they'd be honorable people. . . .

"It's worse than abortion. They took away the right of someone to decide to have children. Losing the ability to choose whether I wanted a family—that was the hardest thing for me to get over."

Robins sent her pretrial interrogatories, but did not move to take her deposition. "They went right to trying to settle, because, I believe, I had a strong case," she said. At the same time, Mary said she did not want to go to trial. She found herself unable to bear the prospect of litigating for two to five more years, "never able to put the pain behind me, wondering when I would have to completely relive the experience in a trial situation. . . . I had had enough pain caused by them. . . .

"A lot of things had been blown apart by the hysterectomy; it was an intensely painful period in my life. I was not emotionally stable because of it and its ramifications. I had lost ten pounds in two days. I wanted to heal myself and I knew I couldn't if I had to dredge everything up. I had already waited two years for the setting of a trial date. Money's fine, but were they going to give me my ovaries back? Like, yes, Your Honor, ladies and gentlemen of the jury, are you going to give me a boy child and a girl child? Maybe for that I would have waited for trial."

In February 1982, Mary settled out of court.

Peggy J. Mample, thirty-two years old when I interviewed her in February, is one of several hundred mothers who conceived while wearing a Dalkon Shield and gave birth prematurely, in the third trimester, to a child with a grave birth defect. She was nineteen when she had Melissa, who has cerebral palsy and will be in a wheelchair for life. "Melissa is very intelligent," she told me. "Her only disability is that she can't walk." At home, the child moves about by crawling, but she attends regular classes in a public elementary school.

Peggy Mample is also among the hundreds of mothers who were themselves physically unharmed, or not seriously harmed, by the Shield while, unknown to them, it attacked their unborn children.

She learned she was pregnant in February 1972. At the time, the medical profession was divided as to the wisdom of removing an IUD from a pregnant woman, and her obstetrician was among the physicians who believed the odds were fifty-fifty that removal of the Shield would induce a miscarriage.

The Robins company, which had made no studies at that time of the IUD's potential to induce premature births or of the possible consequences of such births, was making a soothing promotional claim that it would abandon two years later. As the fetus grew, Robins claimed, the Dalkon Shield would be "pushed gently aside" and no harm would befall either the fetus or the mother. The obstetrician's advice was to leave the Shield in place and go to term, and Peggy agreed. She then gave birth prematurely to Melissa on July 22, 1972.

She had no basis for implicating the Shield until almost nine years later. On April 19, 1981, when she was living in Seattle, the CBS investigative news program "60 Minutes" included a scorching segment on "the disaster of the Dalkon Shield." A friend who saw the television program called to tell her about it and to ask if the IUD she had worn was a Shield. This led her to consult a lawyer and, shortly after, to sue Robins.

Peggy Mample's lawyers, Jane I. Fantel and John J. Davids, argued to the jury that the cerebral palsy was the ultimate result of Robins's false effectiveness claims, of its failure to do studies on the Shield's potential to cause premature births, and of its related failure to investigate the consequences of such births.

Checking around the country before and during the trial, Fantel and Davids found thirty more children of Shield wearers who had been born prematurely in the third trimester with major congenital defects. They told me that Robins initially resisted their demands for data on such children, but finally confirmed the number.

Actually, according to trial testimony by Dr. David A. Eschenbach of the University of Washington, an expert on the adverse effects of IUDs, the total number of such children in the United States was 200 to 300.

The jury awarded $125,000 to Mrs. Mample, but nothing to Melissa, holding that a causal relation had not been established between the Shield and her premature birth and cerebral palsy. Mample then filed a new lawsuit for damages for Melissa. In June 1984, when Melissa was almost twelve, a second jury returned a verdict for her. Although the sum is secret, it was well above an initial offer by Robins to settle for $1.4 million.

Mample now lives in Boise, Idaho. She is still enraged when speaking about the company. "I just think it's absolutely incredible that a large corporation can do this to the American public, using us as guinea pigs," she says. "Needless to say, I don't buy Robins's products any more. . . . I just experienced so many emotions—the anger, the shock, of knowing what large corporations, what *this* corporation, did to my child. . . . It's absolutely incredible that the American public puts up with it, that they don't do something about it."

The anger of the Shield's victims has been fueled by Robins's consistent stonewalling and professions of innocence and ignorance. In the face of several thousand settlements, multimillion-dollar court awards of punitive damages, and its own Shield removal campaign, the claims of innocent ignorance seem incredible, but persist. At a series of depositions taken in 1984 by plaintiffs' lawyer Dale Larson, E. Claiborne Robins swore that he was unable to recall ever have discussed the Shield with his son, E. Claiborne Robins Jr., the company's chief executive officer and president.

"You certainly knew, when you started marketing this device, that pelvic inflammatory disease was a life-threatening disease, did you not?" Larson asked. "I don't know that," Robins testified. "I have never thought of it as life-threatening." Did he know it could destroy fertility?" Maybe I should, but I don't know that," he swore. "I have heard that," he added. "I am not sure where."

Larson drew similar answers from Carl Lunsford. Since 1978, when he became senior vice president for research and development, Lunsford has been in charge of the company's medical department and thus the highest-ranking executive with specific jurisdiction over the Shield's safety. He is a chemist whose involvements with the Shield date back to the premarketing year of 1970.

Lunsford swore he recalled no "expressions of concern" by any company official about PID, and did not remember having "personally wondered" about the toll it was taking. He had not tried to find out how many users died. He had not "personally reviewed" any studies of the Shield's safety or effectiveness in preventing conception. Did he have "any curiosity" about why the company, a few months before, had paid $4.6 million, mostly in punitive damages, to settle seven Shield lawsuits? The answer was "no."

In February 1977, extremely few of the more than 800,000 American women believed to be wearing the Shield had the faintest notion that the devices were becoming more hazardous with each passing day. But Bradley Post, a leading plaintiff's lawyer, did know of the danger, and so he wrote a letter to the company. He asked that Robins mail a corrective "Dear Doctor" letter, partly to urge "immediate removal of devices in use."

Upon receiving no response, Post sent a second letter. He wrote that he had just learned of deaths of two young women, that the circumstances were clearly causally related to their Shields, and that he was concerned about how many more fatalities and serious injuries would have to occur before Robins would take preventive action. No response came to this plea, either.

Four years later, a sequence of deaths began to be reported among long-time Shield users who were not pregnant. The first, in November 1981, was a Los Angeles woman; the second, in April 1983, was Eugenie Standeford, thirty-four, of New Orleans. Ten months later, on February 29, 1984, Judge Lord pleaded for a recall in an instantly famous courtroom reprimand to three senior company officers. He told E. Claiborne Robins Jr., the company's chief executive officer; Carl Lunsford, the senior vice president, and William A. Forrest Jr., the vice president and general counsel:

"The only conceivable reasons you have not recalled this product are that it would hurt your balance sheet and alert women who already have been harmed that you may be liable for their injuries. . . . If this were a case in equity, I would order that your company make an effort to locate each and every person who still wears this device and recall your product. But this court does not have the power to do so. I must therefore resort to moral persuasion and a personal appeal to each of you. . . . You are the corporate conscience. Please, in the name of humanity, lift your eyes above the bottom line. . . . Please, gentlemen, give consideration to tracing down the victims and sparing them the agony that will surely be theirs."

Robins contended, however, that no campaign was needed; because the Shield was no more hazardous than rival IUDs.

Eighteen days after Judge Lord's appeal, Christa Berlin, forty-one, was admitted to the Los Angeles County-University of Southern California Medical Center with lower abdominal pain and fever. The diagnosis was a pelvic abscess. Antibiotics in high doses were injected into her, but her condition worsened, requiring drastic surgery including a hysterectomy. After the operation her condition improved for a time, only to deteriorate again.

"Despite intensive care and cardiorespiratory support," said Dr. Charles M. March, the chief gynecologist, in a letter to the company, "she expired on the eighteenth postoperative day." He pointed out that Berlin had worn a Shield for many years. In October 1984, six months after she died, Robins finally announced a recall campaign. It is reasonable to suggest the Eugenie Standeford, Christa Berlin, and other women might not have died, and that thousands of other women would not have suffered pain and agony, if Robins had acted earlier. But Robins consistently claimed—and continues to claim—that the Dalkon Shield was safe and effective when "properly used."

Robins executives insist that they did not know of any special hazard. But they did know, and they chose to do nothing—until it was much too late.

What does the Dalkon Shield castastrophe teach us? Not that the A.H. Robins company was a renegade in the pharmaceutical industry. Yes, Robins knowingly and willfully put corporate greed before human walfare; suppressed scientific studies that would ascertain safety and effectiveness; concealed hazards from consumers, the medical profession, and government; assigned a lower value to foreign lives than to American lives; behaved ruthlessly toward victims who sued, and hired outside experts who would give accommodating testimony. Yet almost every other major drug company has done one or more of these things, some have done them repeatedly or routinely, and some still continue to do so.

Nor does the Shield catastrophe teach us that the pharmaceutical industry is unique. Cigarette companies profit from smoking, the single greatest cause of preventable disease and death. Knowingly and willfully, automobile manufacturers have sold cars that would become rolling incinerators in rear-end collisions; chemical companies have sold abroad carcinogenic pesticides that are banned here; makers of infant formula have, in impoverished Third World countries, deprived babies of breast milk, the nearly perfect food; assorted industries have dumped poisonous wastes into the environment; coal companies have falsified records showing the exposure of miners to the particles that cause black lung disease; military contractors have supplied defective weapons to the armed services.

No, the lesson of the Dalkon Shield catastrophe is not that Robins alone behaved in an immoral or unexpected fashion, but that, first, the corporate structure itself—oriented as it is toward profit and away from liability—is a standing invitation to such conduct; second, the global scale of contemporary marketing has made hazardous corporate activities more perilous to ever larger numbers of people, and, third, all the deterrents and restraints that normally govern our lives—religion, conscience, criminal codes, economic competition, press exposure, social ostracism—have been overwhelmed.

Government provides insufficient and erratic protection, in part because it is subject to political pressure from both Congress and the corporations themselves, and in part because of the lethargy of entrenched bureaucracy. Thus, despite evidence produced by trial lawyers that rotting tail strings put large numbers of women at risk, the Food and Drug Administration did nothing to protect Shield wearers for nine years, from the time the Shield went off the market in 1974 until 1983, when a study by the Centers for Disease Control incriminated the device.

The FDA never acted on a petition filed by the National Women's Health Network in April 1983 for a recall, to be paid for by Robins, to ensure retrieval of the Shield "from all women who currently wear it" and for imposition of criminal penalties. I am not suggesting that we should abandon Government regulation, but only that we must recognize its limitations. As it stands now, it often provides the illusion, but not the substance, of adequate protection.

Modern society cannot function without the large organization. It manages our great endeavors; it brings us great good. The need today is to stop the individuals who run corporations from inflicting harm. This will not be done by weakening or eliminating existing deterrents and restraints, such as Federal regulators; our hopes lie in strengthening them and adding new ones.

For the foreseeable future, there is no prospect of enacting legislation embodying the powerful moral command in Liviticus 19:16: "Neither shalt thou stand idly by the blood of thy neighbor." Not so long as Ronald Reagan is President. Not so long as the likes of George Bush may succeed him. Not so long as Congress allows special interests to control election financing. And not so long as Americans remain content to live with the paradoxical proposition that harm knowingly and willfully inflicted on them is to be punished, even by death, if done for personal reasons, but is to be unpunished, not even by a day in jail, if done for corporate reasons.

But even in today's political climate, growing numbers of Americans have awakened to the paradox. They have become aware, in part through the repercussions of the Shield disaster, of the impossibility of reconciling personal responsibility with corporate immunity; they know that the proposition is fraudulent. As the public mood becomes more receptive to efforts to hold individuals accountable for corporate actions, we can expect prosecutors, governors, and legislators in many states to make such efforts, and to earn public approval for doing so.

[Only last summer in Illinois, three former executives of Film Recovery Systems, Inc., in Elk Grove Village were successfully prosecuted for murdering a sixty-one-year-old Polish immigrant who had inhaled cyanide used to recover silver from used X-ray film. The murder charges, brought by Cook County prosecutors, were said to be the first in a work-related death. Circuit Judge Ronald J.P. Banks sentenced the executives to twenty-five years in prison and $10,000 fines. Such prosecutions must proliferate, and state officeholders and candidates must make passage of tougher laws an issue.] The press and clergy, too, will have to take the stand that a person's criminal and immoral conduct is criminal, period, and that no ethical counterargument exists.

Judge Lord saw the absurdity of condemning what a man did in a bedroom but not in a boardroom when he said: "We still haven't grasped that the man who assaults women from an office chair is as grave a sinner as the man who assaults a women in an alley." Surely the time has come to extend the definition of immoral conduct into the boardroom and the corporate office.

3 / A Plea for Corporate Conscience

JUDGE MILES W. LORD

Following is the prepared text of the courtroom statement made by Miles W. Lord, Chief U.S. District Judge for Minnesota, on February 29, 1984, to three officers of the A. H. Robins Company who were before him: E. Claiborne Robins, Jr., president and chief executive officer; Carl D. Lunsford, senior vice-president for research and development, and William A. Forrest, Jr., vice-president and general counsel.

Mr. Robins, Mr. Forrest, and Dr. Lunsford: After months of reflection, study, and cogitation—and no small amount of prayer—I have concluded it perfectly appropriate to make to you this statement, which will constitute my plea to you to seek new horizons in corporate consciousness and a new sense of personal responsibility for the activities of those who work under you in the name of the A. H. Robins Company.

It is not enough to say, "I did not know," "It was not me," "Look elsewhere." Time and time again, each of you has used this kind of argument in refusing to acknowledge your responsibility and in pretending to the world that the chief officers and the directors of your gigantic multinational corporation have no responsibility for the company's acts and omissions.

In a speech I gave several years ago (in the document which I have just asked you to read), I suggested to the hundreds of ministers of the gospel who constitute the Minnesota Council of Churches that the accumulation of corporate wrongs is, in my mind, a manifestation of individual sin.

You, Mr. Robins, have been heard to boast many times that the growth and prosperity of this company is a direct result of its having been in the Robins family for three generations. The stamp of the Robins family is upon it. The corporation is built in the image of the Robins mentality.

41

You, Dr. Lunsford, as director of the company's most sensitive and important subdivision, have violated every ethical precept to which every doctor under your supervision must pledge as he gives the oath of Hippocrates and assumes the mantle of one who would help and cure and nurture unto the physical needs of the populace.

You, Mr. Forrest, are a lawyer—one who, upon finding his client in trouble, should counsel and guide him along a course which will comport with the legal, moral, and ethical principles which must bind us all. You have not brought honor to your profession, Mr. Forrest.

Gentlemen, the results of these activities and attitudes on your part have been catastrophic. Today as you sit here attempting once more to extricate yourselves from the legal consequences of your acts, none of you has faced up to the fact that more than nine thousand women have made claims that they gave up part of their womanhood so that your company might prosper. It is alleged that others gave their lives so you might so prosper. And there stand behind them legions more who have been injured but who have not sought relief in the courts of this land.

I dread to think what would have been the consequences if your victims had been men rather than women, women who seem through some strange quirk of our society's mores to be expected to suffer pain, shame, and humiliation.

If one poor young man were, by some act of his—without authority or consent—to inflict such damage upon one woman, he would be jailed for a good portion of the rest of his life. And yet your company, without warning to women, invaded their bodies by the millions and caused them injuries by the thousands. And when the time came for these women to make their claims against your company, you attacked their characters. You inquired into their sexual practices and into the identity of their sex partners. You exposed these women—and ruined families and reputations and careers—in order to intimidate those who would raise their voices against you. You introduced issues that had no relationship whatsoever to the fact that you planted in the bodies of these women instruments of death, of mutilation, of disease.

I wish to make it absolutely clear that I am specifically directing and limiting my remarks to that which I have learned and observed in these consolidated cases before me. If an incident arises involving another product made by the A. H. Robins Company, an independent judgment would have to be made as to the conduct of your company concerning that product. Likewise, a product made by any other company must be judged upon the individual facts of that case.

Gentlemen, you state that your company has suffered enough, that the infliction of further punishment in the form of punitive damages will cause harm to your ongoing business, will punish innocent shareholders, and could conceivably depress your profits to the point where you could not survive as a competitor in this industry. When the poor and downtrodden in this country commit crimes, they too plead that these are crimes of survival and that they should be excused for illegal acts which helped them escape desperate economic straits. On a few occasions when these excuses are made and a contrite and remorseful defendant promises to mend his ways, courts will give heed to such a plea. But no court would heed this plea when the individual denies the wrongful nature of his deeds and gives no indication that he will mend his ways. Your company, in the face of overwhelming evidence, denies its guilt and continues its monstrous mischief.

Mr. Forrest, you have told me that you are working with members of the Congress of the United States to ask them to find a way of forgiving you from punitive damages which might otherwise be imposed. Yet the profits of your company continue to mount. Your last financial report boasts of new records for sales and earnings, with a profit of more than $58 million in 1983. And all the while, insofar as this court is able to determine, you three men and your company still engage in the selfsame course of wrongdoing in which you originally commenced. Until such time as your company indicates that it is willing to cease and desist this deception and to seek out and advise victims, your remonstrances to Congress and to the courts of this country are indeed hollow and cynical. The company has not suffered, nor have you men personally. You are collectively being enriched by millions of dollars each year. There is as yet no evidence that your company has suffered any penalty whatsoever from these litigations. In fact, the evidence is to the contrary.

The case law indicates that the purpose of punitive damages is to make an award which will punish a defendant for his wrongdoing. Punishment traditionally involves the principles of revenge, rehabilitation, and deterrence. There is no evidence I have been able to find in my review of these cases to indicate that any one of these factors have been accomplished.

Mr. Robins, Mr. Forrest, Dr. Lunsford: You have not been rehabilitated. Under your direction, your company has in fact continued to allow women, tens of thousands of them, to wear this device—a deadly depth charge in their wombs, ready to explode at any time. Your attorney, Mr. Alexander Slaughter, denies that tens of thousands of these devices are still in the bodies of women. But I submit to you that Mr. Slaughter has no more basis for his denial than the plaintiffs have for stating it as truth, because we simply do not know how many women are still wearing these devices, and your company is not willing to find out. The only conceivable reasons you have not recalled this product are that it would hurt your balance sheet and alert women who already have been harmed that you may be liable for their injuries. You have taken the bottom line as your guiding beacon, and the low road as your route. This is corporate irresponsibility at its meanest. Rehabilitation involves an admission of guilt, a certain contrition, an acknowledgment of wrongdoing, and a resolution to take a new course toward a better life. I find none of this in the instance of you and your corporation. Confession is good for the soul, gentlemen. Face up to your misdeeds. Acknowledge the personal responsibility that you have for the activities of those who work under you. Rectify this evil situation. Warn the potential future victims and recompense those who already have been harmed.

Mr. Robins, Mr. Forrest, Dr. Lunsford: I see little in the history of this case that would deter others from partaking of like acts. The policy of delay and obfuscation practiced by your lawyers in courts throughout this country has made it possible for you and your insurance company, Aetna Casualty and Surety Company, to delay the payment of these claims for such a long period that the interest you earn in the interim covers the cost of these cases. You, in essence, pay nothing out of your pocket to settle these cases. What other corporate officials could possibly learn a lesson from this? The only lesson could be that it pays to delay compensating victims and to intimidate, harass, and shame the injured parties.

Mr. Robins, Mr. Forrest, Dr. Lunsford: You gentlemen have consistently denied any knowledge of the deeds of the company you control. Mr. Robins, I have read your deposition. Many times you state that your management style was such as to delegate work and responsibility to other employees in matters involving the most important aspects of this nation's health. Judge Frank Theis, who presided over the discovery of these cases during the multidistrict litigation proceedings, noted this phenomenon in a recent opinion. He wrote, "The project manager for Dalkon Shield explains that a particular question should have gone to the medical department, the medical department representative explains that the question was really the bailiwick of the quality-control department, and the quality-control department representative explains that the project manager was the one with the authority to make a decision on that question." Under these circumstances, Judge Theis noted, "it is not at all unusual for the hard questions posed in Dalkon Shield cases to be unanswerable by anyone from Robins."

Your company seeks to segment and fragment the litigation of these cases nationwide. The courts of this country are now burdened with more than three thousand Dalkon Shield cases. The sheer number of claims and the dilatory tactics used by your company's attorneys clog court calendars and consume vast amounts of judicial and jury time. Your company settles those cases in which it finds itself in an uncomfortable position, a handy device for avoiding any proceeding which would give continuity or cohesiveness to this nationwide problem. The decision as to which cases to try rests almost solely at the whim and discretion of the A. H. Robins Company. In order that no plaintiff or group of plaintiffs might assert a sustained assault upon your system of evasion and avoidance, you time after time demand that able lawyers who have knowledge of the facts must, as a price of settling their cases, agree to never again take a Dalkon Shield case nor to help any less experienced lawyers with their cases against your company.

Minnesota lawyers have filed cases in this jurisdiction for women from throughout the United States. The cases of these women have waited on the calendar of this court for as many as three years. The evidence they will present at trial is predominantly generic evidence concerning the company's actions, which is as easy to produce in Minnesota as anywhere else. Yet your company's attorneys persist in asking that these cases be transferred to other jurisdictions and to other judges unfamiliar with the cases, there to wait at the bottom of the calendars for additional months and years before they have their day in court.

Another of your callous legal tactics is to force women of little means to withstand the onslaught of your well-financed, nationwide team of attorneys, and to default if they cannot keep pace. You target your worst tactics for the meek and the poor.

(I should point out that the Faegre & Benson law firm, local counsel for your company in the consolidated cases before me, has a high reputation for fair play, integrity, and fidelity to the court. Faegre & Benson, and other local firms retained for trials across the country, are not responsible for the overall strategic decisions of your company.)

Despite your company's protestations, it is evident that these thousands of cases cannot be viewed in isolation, one at a time. The multidistrict litigation panel of the federal court system found these cases to have sufficient similarity on issues of fact and law to warrant their reference to a single judge who, for varying periods of time, conducted discovery, depositions, and proceedings designed to devise an efficient method of handling these cases. In each of these thousands of cases, the focal point of the inquiry is the same: the conduct of your company through its acts and omissions. Indeed, Judge Gerald Heaney of the Court of Appeals for the Eighth Circuit recently urged judges in Minnesota to work together to devise a coordinated system for dealing with all of their Dalkon Shield cases.

These litigations must be viewed as a whole. Were these women to be gathered together with their injuries in one location, this would be denominated a disaster of the highest magnitude. The mere fact that these women are separated by geography blurs the total picture. Here we have thousands of victims, present and potential, whose injuries arise from the same series of operative facts. You have made no effort whatsoever to locate them and bring them together to seek a common solution to their plight.

If this were a case in equity, I would order that your company make an effort to locate each and every woman who still wears this device and recall your product. But this court does not have the power to do so. I must therefore resort to moral persuasion and a personal appeal to each of you. Mr. Robins, Mr. Forrest, and Dr. Lunsford: You are the people with the power to recall. You are the corporate conscience.

Please, in the name of humanity, lift your eyes above the bottom line. You, the men in charge, must surely have hearts and souls and consciences. If the thought of facing up to your transgressions is so unbearable to you, you might do as Roger Tuttle did and confess to your Maker, beg forgiveness, and mend your ways.

Please, gentlemen, give consideration to tracing down the victims and sparing them the agony that will surely be theirs.

4 / The Dumping of Hazardous Products on Foreign Markets

MARK DOWIE and *MOTHER JONES*

Tom Mboya was the hope of the western world. Bright, energetic, popular and inclined to be democratic—he was a born leader who, Washington hoped, would rise to power in Kenya and help keep Africa safe for United States commerce. In 1969 he was shot down in the streets of Nairobi. An emergency rescue squad was by his side in minutes. They plugged him into the latest gadget in resuscitative technology—a brand new U.S. export called the Res-Q-Aire. What the rescue team didn't know as they watched Tom Mboya's life slip away was that this marvelous device had been recalled from the American market by the U.S. government because it was found to be totally ineffective. The patient died.

Losing Mboya to the Res-Q-Aire was perhaps a subtle retribution for the U.S. for to this day we allow our business leaders to sell, mostly to Third World nations, shiploads of defective medical devices, lethal drugs, known carcinogens, toxic pesticides, contaminated foods and other products found unfit for American consumption.

Ten years after Mboya's assassination, in fact, Kenya itself remains a major market for unsafe, ineffective and contaminated American products. At the 1977 meeting of the United Nations Environmental Program, Kenya Minister of Water Development Dr. D. J. Kiano warned that developing nations would no longer tolerate being used as "dumping grounds for products that have not been adequately tested" and that their people should not be used as "guinea pigs" for chemicals.

The prevailing sentiment in Washington contrasts considerably with Dr. Kiano's. Say the word "dumping" in federal government

47

circles and the predominant response will be "Oh, yes, 'dumping.' Really must be stopped. It's outrageous, not in our economic interests at all . . . unscrupulous bastards. . . ."

Sounds as if we've solved the problem, doesn't it, except what our bureaucrats are talking about, one discovers, is foreign corporations "dumping" low-priced goods on the American market—Japanese cars, Taiwanese televisions, Hong Kong stereos, Australian beef, etc. The export of banned and hazardous products, which is a more lethal form of "dumping," is considered business as usual. Dumping is, in fact, *big* business as usual. It involves not only manufacturers and retailers, a vast array of export brokers, tramp steamers, black marketeers and go-betweens who traffic an estimated $1.2 billion worth of unsafe goods overseas every year, but also the United States Export-Import Bank, which finances large dumps; the Commerce, State and Treasury Departments, which have the statutory authority to stop or control dumping, but won't; and a President who, in his quiet way, subverts the efforts of the few progressive members of Congress who seek to pass uniform anti-dumping legislation.

Occasionally, a particularly scandalous dump will come to the attention of conscientious Americans. Most dumps, however, are performed quietly, the product moving unnoticed in the fast flow of normal trade between nations. And dumping is not limited to chemicals and consumer products. When a firm's production facilities and industrial equipment are condemned by the Occupational Safety and Health Administration, the manufacturer often simply closes up shop and moves the factory to Mexico or Jamaica, where occupational health standards are virtually nonexistent. Even entire technologies are dumped. Nuclear power, which seems certain to receive a "hazardous" classification before long in the U.S., is today being dumped on energy-starved nations like the Philippines and India.

We are only beginning to discover how toxic and carcinogenic are some of the chemicals we use, chemicals with the potential to affect the entire global environment and human gene pool. Moreover, the number of other consumer products that maim or kill shows no sign of diminishing. The list of banned and hazardous products is thus bound to grow, which *should* making dumping a major international issue for the 1980s.

Although the bottom line motive is always profit, hazardous products are dumped to solve different problems. For nonmanufacturers—wholesalers, retailers, brokers, importers and exporters—the problem is generally just a matter of inventory. Salvation often comes in the form of a broker, offering to buy the banned goods at a "closeout" price for resale in an unnamed (read, Third World) market.

It's not that simple, however, for manufacturers who have invested capital in tools, dies, assembly plants, personnel, machines and land. When a company like A. H. Robins foresees the withdrawal of a product like the Dalkon Shield intrauterine device, it dumps a million units on foreign countries, voluntarily withdraws the product and closes up shop. The company takes a small loss buying back recalled inventory (which it writes off), and its capital investment is amortized.

It was Tris that brought dumping into the political arena. Tris (2, 3-dibromopropyl) phosphate is a fire-retardant chemical used to treat synthetic flammable fabrics. In June of 1977, after Tris was found to cause cancer in animals, millions of pairs of infant pajamas and tons of children's sleepwear were suddenly withdrawn from the U.S. market by the Consumer Product Safety Commission (CPSC). When some of the manufacturers, stuck with huge repurchased inventories of these carcinogenic garments, threatened to dump them on the overseas markets, the CPSC claimed that it had no statutory authority to stop them from doing so. In fact, although the CPSC, the EPA and the FDA together have removed over 500 pesticides, drugs and consumer products from the American market for health, safety or environmental reasons, the patchwork of regulations obfuscates what limited power these agencies have to prohibit the export of dangerous products.

When President Carter, who had the authority to stop dumping with a simple Executive Order, learned of the Tris situation, he authorized the formation of an Interagency Working Group to develop a uniform national policy on dumping. Although such task forces can provide a valuable forum for intra-government communication and often make important policy recommendations, the Interagency Working Group on Hazardous Substances Export Policy (HSEP)—chaired by Carter's Special Assistant for Consumer Affairs, Esther Peterson—is, in fact, being used to table the issue until our balance of trade improves. Dumping, you see, is exporting; and although banned and hazardous products represent only about one percent of our total trade, every percent seems to count when we are constantly running a trade deficit of over $25 billion a year.

Dumpers have proven themselves to be a highly imaginative lot. Here are a few of their methods to circumvent regulatory agencies at home and suspicious importers abroad:

The Name Change: When a product is withdrawn from the American market, receiving a lot of bad publicity in the process, the astute dumper simply changes its name.

The Last Minute Pullout: When it looks as if a chemical being tested by the Environmental Protection Agency won't pass, the manufacturer will withdraw the application for registration and then label the chemical "for export only." That way, the manufacturer doesn't have to notify the importing country that the chemical is banned in the U.S.

Dump the Whole Factory: Many companies, particularly pesticide manufacturers, will simply close down their American plants and begin manufacturing a hazardous product in a country close to a good market.

The Formula Change: A favorite with drug and pesticide companies. Changing a formula slightly by adding or subtracting an inert ingredient prevents detection by spectrometers and other scanning devices keyed to certain molecular structures.

The Skip: Brazil—a prime drug market with its large population and virulent tropical diseases—has a law that says no one may import a drug that is not approved for use in the country of origin. A real challenge for the wily dumper. How does he do it?

Guatemala has no such law; in fact, Guatemala spends very little each year regulating drugs. So, the drug is first shipped to Guatemala, which becomes the export nation.

The Ingredient Dump: Your product winds up being banned. Don't dump it. Some reporter will find a bill of lading and expose you. Export the ingredients separately—perhaps via different routes—to a small recombining facility or assembly plant you have set up where you're dumping it, or in a country along the way. Reassemble them and dump the product.

The contraceptive double standard surfaced as a public issue only in the summer of 1978, when a congressional committee held hearings on the Depo-Provera problem: Should the U.S. government subsidize the export to Third World nations of a contraceptive drug that had been ruled unsafe for American women? Pharmaceutical company spokespeople, officials of the U.S. Agency for International Development (AID) and representatives of private population control agencies stood up one after another to advance the "humanitarian" defense of the double standard. Because the risks of dying in childbirth are so much greater in the Third World than in the United States, they asserted, the use of almost any contraceptive is justified. Scientists from selected Third World governments, many of them U.S.-sponsored dictatorships like Chile and Thailand, seconded the argument, adding that their "national sovereignty" would be violated if they were denied access to the contraceptive of their choice. Consumer representatives countered that there is no excuse for sending our *least* safe contraceptive abroad and questioned the accountability of the "sovereign" governments, which it is now known, have received millions of dollars in bribes from U.S. drug companies like Upjohn Co. (maker of Depo-Provera) and G. D. Searle Co. (a manufacturer of birth control pills).

The contraceptive issue is no different than the case of Tris-treated pajamas, carcinogenic pesticides or lethal antibiotics: products that had been found unsafe for domestic use are still being sold overseas. There is, however, a crucial difference in the case of contraceptives: dumping them is not only a common business practice; it is part of U.S. foreign policy.

The dangers of the Dalkon Shield IUD were well known before the dump began in 1972. Only a few months after the Dalkon Shield went on the market in 1971, reports of adverse reactions began pouring into the headquarters of the manufacturer, A. H. Robins Co. There were cases of pelvic inflammatory disease (an infection of the uterus that can require weeks of bed rest and antibiotic treatment), septicemia (blood poisoning), pregnancies resulting in spontaneous abortions, ectopic (tubal) pregnancies and perforations in the uterus. In a number of cases, the damage was so severe as to require a hysterectomy. There were even medical reports of Dalkon Shields ripping their way through the walls of the uterus and being found floating free in the abdominal cavity far from the uterus. According to a recent and probably conservative U.S. medical estimate, the Dalkon Shield caused over 200,000 cases of serious uterine infections in this country alone. For every million dollars in profit the manufacturer has made on the Shield, U.S. women—those who could afford medical care at all—spent an estimated $20 million for medical care on problems arising from its use.

After the Dalkon Shield intrauterine device killed at least 17 women in the United States, the manufacturer withdrew it from the domestic market. It was sold overseas after the American recall and is still in common use in some countries.

Depo-Provera, an injectable contraceptive banned for such use in the United States because it caused malignant tumors in beagles and monkeys, is sold by the Upjohn Co. in 70 other countries, where it is widely used in U.S.-sponsored population control programs.

For 11 years, starting in 1967, Upjohn battled to get FDA approval for Depo-Provera. But in 1971, after studies done on beagle dogs showed that Depo was carcinogenic in high doses, the FDA was alarmed enough to call a halt to all clinical test of the drug. On March 7, 1978, the FDA sent Upjohn a letter notifying the company of its final decision: Depo-Provera was "not approvable" for use in the U.S.

Domestic criticism of Depo-Provera has not prevented a plentiful supply from reaching the Third World. The FDA's refusal to approve

Depo only meant that Upjohn could not ship the drug from its U.S. plants. It could, however, ship the drug from its Belgian subsidiary to whatever foreign commercial outlets it could find.

It has found plenty. In Belize, Central America, Depo is freely available at drugstores, despite what our correspondent reports as "many instances of amenorrhea (lack of menstrual periods) or profuse bleeding." A letter from Guatemala City to the Washington-based National Women's Health Network, related that in Honduras, El Salvador, Costa Rica, Nicaragua, Panama and the Dominican Republic "it is completely possible to buy it over the counter with no prescription."

This, apparently, is not enough for some parties. AID would like to be able to buy up huge batches of Depo at bulk rates, and Upjohn would like nothing better. Both testified to that effect to the U.S. Congress. An AID-subsidized dump could mean a four-fold increase in Upjohn's Depo sales.

There are several ways this could happen. First, AID could simply buy Depo from Upjohn's Belgian subsidiary and ship from there, as it has threatened to do. Another possibility is that Congress could pass a new drug reform act allowing for the export of nonapproved drugs. (A bill that may liberalize drug exports was approved by the Senate in September 1979). Or, the FDA could reverse its position on Depo-Provera and approve it for use in the United States, though perhaps only for special subgroups (the mentally retarded and drug addicts have been proposed). This, believe it or not, is a real possibility.

Dumping pesticides is a little different than selling Dalkon Shields or Tris-soaked pajamas to unsuspecting consumers. Heinous as those dumps might be, the injury or death inflicted as a result happens on an individual basis, in distinct tragedies, one body at a time. Not so with pesticides. Most of the peasants applying the poisons to crops can read neither the English nor the Spanish instructions printed on the labels of the chemical containers. Pesticides are often poured on crops in excessive amounts. Many people, in addition to the pests, are poisoned by the chemicals—about 500,000 yearly, according to the World Health Organization. Some victims die immediately; the long-term effects on the rest are unknown.

"The people who work in the fields of Central America are treated like half humans," says Dr. Lou Falcon, a University of California entomologist who visits the region often. "When an airplane flies over to spray, they can leave if they want, but they won't be paid their seven cents a day, or whatever. They often live in huts in the middle of the fields. Their homes, their children and their food get contaminated."

Pesticide poisoning is only one aspect of the massive dumping of these chemicals. A three-month investigation by us and the Center for

Investigative Reporting shows that U.S. companies—while not the worst offenders, since that distinction belongs to firms headquartered in Europe—have an enormous stake in exporting these chemicals. Uncontrolled, the worldwide pesticide trade is on its way to becoming a scandal of international proportions:

- Nearly 40 percent of the 1.6 billion pounds of pesticides sold annually in this country is sold to export buyers. It appears that every pesticide banned or restricted by the federal government here has been exported. A full 15 percent of U.S. pesticide exports are "unregistered." They are chemicals that were never licensed, tested or reviewed by the EPA at all.
- Pesticides are sold throughout the Third World without controls to people who usually do not know how the chemicals should be safely used. Leptophos, a nerve-damaging pesticide that brings on paralysis in its victims, was never approved for sale in the U.S. In Indonesia, according to an official of that country's Food and Agriculture Organization, leptophos was sold "alongside the potatoes and rice . . . people just collect it in sugar sacks, milk cartons, Coke bottles. . . ."
- Both farmworkers themselves and those who eat food grown throughout the developing world with the aid of pesticides run a high risk of pesticide poisoning. One Central American farm survey found the levels of the pesticide aldrin on cabbage to be nearly 2,000 times the level allowed in food sold in the U.S. The average content of DDT in the blood of people in Guatemala and Nicaragua was over 30 times the U.S. average.
- Not only are U.S.-based companies selling pesticides overseas, they also are buying them there. In Costa Rica, the main importer for seven heavily restricted U.S. pesticides (DDT, aldrin, dieldrin, heptachlor, chlordane, endrin and BHC) is not a local farming operation, but Ortho, a division of Chevron Chemical Co.—an arm of Standard Oil of California. This way, the multinational companies circumvent U.S. regulations and continue using hazardous chemicals for food production.
- The "vast majority" of the nearly one billion pounds of pesticides used each year in the Third World is applied to crops that are then exported back to the U.S. and other rich countries, according to WHO. This fact undercuts the industry's main argument defending pesticide dumping. "We see nothing wrong with helping the hungry world eat," is the way a Velsicol Chemical Company executive puts it. Yet, the entire dumping process bypasses the local population's need for food.

The hazards of dumping pesticides overseas are many, but it would be inaccurate to believe they are the Third World's alone. Pesticides, once dumped, have a way of coming back, like a boomerang. U.S. government spot checks have found that approximately 10 percent of imported food is contaminated with illegal levels of pesticides. The Food and Drug Administration (FDA) reports that half of the green coffee beans imported by this country are contaminated with pesticides that have been previously banned in the U.S. At least 20 pesticides, potential carcinogens, are undetectable with FDA tests used to find residues in food. In many other cases, the FDA simply does not know what the substances are that do show up in its tests.

There are, for example 94 different pesticides used by the six coffee-growing countries in Central and South America. Studies by the General Accounting Office, Congress's investigative arm, found that, of those, 64 are not detectable by FDA multiresidue tests. Of those that are detectable, only 18 have tolerance levels set for restricting the sale of coffee contaminated with them. This means that imported coffee can be sold in the U. S. with the residues of 76 pesticides that are either undetectable or completely unregulated.

Chloramphenicol is one of the "wonder" drugs, an antibiotic effective against a broad range of infections. However, it has equally powerful side effects. One of them is aplastic anemia, a frequently fatal blood disease. Extrapolating from fatality-rate figures given by the California State Department of Health, we can estimate that between 888 and 1,487 Americans have died from aplastic anemia induced by chloramphenicol. The drug is marketed in this country by Parke, Davis & Company, most commonly under the name Chloromycetin.

Despite this risk, chloramphenicol still is uniquely effective against certain esoteric diseases, one of them being typhoid fever. The problem (for the drug companies) is that there are only a few hundred cases of typhoid fever a year in the U. S. Hence, Parke, Davis, for many years aggressively pushed its Chloromycetin as a cure for a wide variety of other maladies. Experts testifying some years ago before Senator Gaylord Nelson's Small Business Subcommitttee on Monopoly said that between 90 and 99 percent of Chloromycetin prescriptions were being given out for common colds, acne or other conditions for which no drugs are effective or other drugs are safer.

Eventually, under pressure of congressional hearings, lawsuits and other publicity, chloramphenicol sales in the U. S. declined sharply. Parke, Davis began printing warnings on Chloromycetin packages sold in the U. S. stressing the drug should only be used for a few life-threatening illnesses. Are these warnings "justifiable?" Senator Nelson asked Parke, Davis executive Leslie Lueck at a 1967 hearing. "Yes," he replied. To Lueck's consternation, Nelson then produced an ad for Chloromycetin from the British medical journal *The Lancet* that carried no warnings at all. Lueck made some excuses; Nelson said: "I don't see how you people can sleep at night."

If Parke, Davis people lost any sleep over Britain, they ought to have become insomniacs over Latin America. There, University of California pharmacologist Dr. Milton Silverman reported in a 1976 study, chloramphenicol was recommended to physicians for treatment of all sorts of conditions—including tonsillitis and bronchitis—that were scarcely life-threatening. Parke, Davis gave no warnings at all about the drug to doctors in Guatemala. Costa Rica and a rival supplier of chloramphenicol recommended its brand for whooping cough; and while it disclosed a few hazards to doctors in Central America, it listed none at all in Colombia and Ecuador.

Besides causing an unknown number of deaths from aplastic anemia, promiscuous use of chloramphenicol—like that of many antibiotics—has had a more serious consequence: bacteria have built up resistance to it.

No one knew how serious a problem this would be until a 1972–73 epidemic of typhoid fever in Mexico. Believed to be the most catastrophic outbreak of typhoid in history, it afflicted about 100,000 people. Up until this point, most doctors had assumed that chloramphenicol would prove as effective against typhoid as it had in the past. To their dismay, they were wrong. The particular typhoid bacteria they were dealing with had, through long exposure, built up resistance to chloramphenicol. Doctors were largely helpless; 20,000 of the typhoid victims died.

The liberal compromise on the dumping issue is notification. Invoking the principles of national sovereignty, self-determination and free trade, government officials and legislators have devised a system whereby foreign governments are notified whenever a product is banned, deregulated, suspended or cancelled by an American regulatory agency. The notification system is handled by the State Department, whose policy statement on the subject reads in part, "No country should establish itself as the arbiter of others' health and safety standards. Individual governments are generally in the best position to establish standards of public health and safety."

The main problem with notification is the logic behind it. Other governments are generally not in a position to establish safety standards, let alone control imports into their countries. In fact, the countries where most of our banned and hazardous products are dumped lack regulatory agencies, testing laboratories or well-staffed customs departments. In 1978, Nigeria's Environmental Protection

Ministry was one person. He recently told the U. S. EPA that it didn't matter whether or not he was notified when a pesticide was suspended; there was nothing he could do to stop its importation.

When our EPA, FDA or CPSC finds a product to be hazardous, they notify our State Department as required or as a matter of protocol. State, which we have found to be no opponent of dumping, is then supposed to send a communique to each American embassy overseas. Each embassy is, in turn, supposed to notify the appropriate foreign officials. However, the Commerce, Consumer and Monetary Affairs Subcommittee of the House Committee on Government Operations discovered in hearings held in July of 1978 that the agencies frequently neglected to inform the State Department when they banned a product. For example, the EPA failed to notify State after suspending such notorious pesticides as kepone, chlordane and heptachlor. The General Accounting Office (GAO) also discovered and testified to the same subcommittee that even when the agencies did notify State, the communiques rarely went further than the U. S. embassies overseas—they almost never reached the foreign officials who might have been able to warn foreign buyers or intercept shipments. One embassy official even admitted to the GAO that he "did not routinely forward notification of chemicals not registered in the host country because it may adversely affect U. S. exporting." The GAO would not tell us the name of location of the official they quoted, but said the sentiment was not unusual.

Some of the foreign officials who have been notified have complained that the communiques are vague and ambiguous, or else so highly technical that they are incomprehensible. Of course, even if clear notification about a product were to reach officials in an importing nation, there is nothing to stop the exporters from changing a product's brand name before they ship.

Perhaps the only aspect of the whole dumping travesty that has kept the issue alive in Washington is reimportation. Members of Congress and bureaucrats who would otherwise ignore or even encourage dumping become irate upon learning that a hazardous product is being reimported (smuggled) into the U. S. for sale, or that an imported fruit or vegetable contains residue of a pesticide long since suspended for American use. Even Esther Peterson, in a memo to President Carter, expressed concern about reimportation.

Remember, it is perfectly legal to dump hazardous products abroad. There are, however, strict measures to prevent reimportation. The FDA allows manufacturers to export banned drugs, staledated drugs and even unapproved new drugs if they are shipped under "an investigational protocol" (for experimentation on other people). But one of the stipulations for the export of drugs removed from the American marketplace is that they never be offered for domestic sale again.

The CPSC, however, can prohibit the export of goods forced off the American market. It can also stop exports that present "an unreasonable risk to persons in the U. S." (through their reimportation, for example), but the CPSC admits that proving unreasonable risk is "very difficult."

The White House Office of Consumer Affairs remains confident that a uniform policy on the export of banned and hazardous products will protect foreign consumers. Our investigations, however, indicate that the corporate dumping urge is rooted in a criminal mentality and that dumpers will, as they already have, find new ways to circumvent whatever legal and regulatory barriers stand between their warehouses and profitable markets for their deadly goods.

Global corporations, with their worldwide network of subsidiaries, high technology and marketing systems, far outstrip the puny regulatory efforts of a government that considers corporate crime a minor nuisance at worst. Nothing short of a complete moral transformation of the corporate ethos will stop dumping. Until that unlikely transformation takes place, we recommend the following:

- Dumping must be clearly defined by statute, and one term, such as "illegal for export," should be applied to American products found to be too dangerous for use here and, hence, anywhere. We should recognize that there are a few—a very few—products that are unsafe for use in the U. S. for which the benefits far outweigh the risks in other countries—for example, certain drugs used to treat tropical diseases or pesticides used to kill the malaria-carrying mosquito. In such cases, when the foreign government is apprised of the risk, the products should be cleared for export to that country only.
- Dumping should be made a criminal offense.
- The government, which already controls exports through the Community Control List and the Bureau of Census (where all exports of over $250 are registered), must accept the responsibility of monitoring the outflow of banned and hazardous products. This responsibility should be taken from the Department of Commerce, where it represents an untenable conflict of interest.
- Notification of product bans, suspensions, cancellations and withdrawals from registration should be made *directly* by the U. S. regulatory agencies to appropriate foreign officials, in language that can be understood.

- The State Department should be relieved of any antidumping responsibility, since it has so deliberately failed to coordinate an effective notification program.

Until all of the above are accomplished, the President should use his powers to stop dumping immediately.

Executives in major exporting corporations argue that if the export of banned and hazardous products is prohibited by statute or Executive Order, foreign buyers will merely turn to European or other suppliers, as they have in the past for weapons and ammunition. Other developed nations do dump; Germany dumps at least as many toxic pesticides as the U. S., and no nation on earth can match Switzerland for dumping baby formula. However, the assumption that foreign buyers will import known toxins and recognized lethal products from one country when they can't get them from another is patently ridiculous.

American business leaders, who tout themselves as the most ethical businesspeople in the world, should lead the way in ending dumping worldwide. It's in their best interest to do so, for by dumping toxins on the Third World they are actually poisoning the very markets they seek to develop.

Additional Readings

Braithwaite, John. *Corporate Crime in the Pharmaceutical Industry*. London: Routledge & Kegan Paul, 1984.

Claybrook, Joan and the Staff of Public Citizen. *Retreat from Safety: Reagan's Attack on America's Health*. New York: Pantheon, 1984.

Cullen, Francis T., Wiliam J. Maakestad, and Gray Cavender. *Corporate Crime Under Attack: The Ford Pinto Case and Beyond*. Cincinnati: Anderson Publishing Co., 1987.

Dowie, Mark et al. "The Illusion of Safety." *Mother Jones*, June 1982, pp. 37–48.

Eddy, Paul, Elaine Potter, and Bruce Page. *Destination Disaster—from the Tri–Motor to the DC–10: The Risks of Flying*. New York: Quadrangle, 1976.

Frank, Nancy. *Crimes Against Health and Safety*. New York: Harrow and Heston, 1985.

Hochstedler, Ellen, ed. *Corporations as Criminals*. Beverly Hills, Calif.: Sage Publications, Inc., 1984.

Knightley, Phillip et al. *Suffer the Children: The Story of Thalidomide*. New York: Viking, 1979.

Margulies, Leah. "Babies, Bottles and Breast Milk: The Nestlé Syndrome." In *The Big Business Reader: On Corporate America*, edited by Mark Green, rev. ed. New York: Pilgrim Press, 1983.

Mintz, Morton. *At Any Cost: Corporate Greed, Women, and the Dalkon Shield*. New York: Pantheon Books Inc., 1985.

Riley, Tom. *The Price of a Life: One Woman's Death from Toxic Shock*. Bethesda, Md.: Adler and Adler, 1986.

Silverman, Milton, Philip R. Lee, and Mia Lydecker. *Prescriptions for Death: The Drugging of the Third World*. Berkeley: University of California Press, 1982.

Simon, David R. and D. Stanley Eitzen. "Corporate Deviance: Human Jeopardy." Chap. 4 in *Elite Deviance*, 2d ed. Boston: Allyn and Bacon, 1986.

Strobel, Lee Patrick. *Reckless Homicide? Ford's Pinto Trial*. South Bend, Ind.: And Books, 1980.

Part II

Injury and Death
in the Workplace

M ARK REUTTER, an investigative journalist and historian, describes a persistent pattern of fatalities and injuries among workers at the Bethelehem Steel Corporation plant at Sparrows Point, Maryland, in his article "The Invisible Risk." Challenging the company's contention that frequent accidents that maim and kill workers are inevitable in view of the dangerous nature of work in the steel industry, Reutter documents the negligence of management in failing to take elementary safety precautions, using hazardous machinery that frequently breaks down, and ignoring clearly dangerous work conditions. Indeed, throughout the steel industry the author argues, the attempt to speed up production with aging machinery has produced an extremely high injury toll that is mostly invisible to the outside world. As Reutter points out, "safety does not necessarily pay." Although the Occupational Safety and Health Administration and state regulatory agencies have convicted steel manufacturers for numerous safety violations, the small fines (rarely exceeding $10,000 for a worker's death) and the negligible costs of workmen's compensation offer few economic incentives to provide a safer work environment—especially when "overhead business expenses" can be absorbed into the price of the steel product.

In "Death by Cotton Dust," an original article written for this anthology, political scientist Richard Guarasci of St. Lawrence University presents several poignant vignettes of workers who are permanently disabled after years of inhaling cotton dust particles in the textile mills of the Carolinas. Guarasci provides an insightful analysis of textile industry politics in southeastern United States, and the failure of OSHA to fulfill the congressional mandate to provide a safe and healthy environment for American workers. Using the cotton industry as a case study in corporate negligence and social injustice, the author describes the oppressive managerial style of large textile manufacturers such as J. P. Stevens—a notorious law violator—many of whose workers have had their lives tragically cut short from the illness known as byssinosis or "brown lung," a disease that slowly and painfully restricts the worker's ability to breathe.

A series of explosions in the Scotia coal mine under Big Black Mountain in Kentucky, which killed 26 miners, is the setting for Harry Caudill's angry indictment of the complacent attitude of company officials and government bureaucrats toward coal mine safety in the Appalachian mining states. Caudill, who is a lawyer and author of several books on the Appalachian region, describes the haphazard practices and flagrant violations of safety regulations at the Scotia mine where production and profit take priority over the lives of the miners who dig out the coal. Although the 26 miners died "under circumstances that reek of carelessness, lack of skill, illegality, incompetence and official neglect," no significant changes have yet occurred in the supervisory personnel and operations of the Scotia mine in the aftermath of this tragedy; no employees of either the coal company or the federal Mine Enforcement and Safety Administration have been indicted or punished for their role in this humanly created disaster.

The final article in this section, "Murder in the Workplace," discusses the unprecedented conviction in 1985 of three executives of Film Recovery Systems, Inc., each sentenced to twenty-five years in prison for their indifference to and tolerance of unsafe working conditions that resulted in the death of a Polish immigrant from cyanide poisoning. Sociologist Nancy Frank describes the Film Recovery Systems plant in which illegal aliens were used as workers, but were not told that the cyanide solution in which they soaked used photographic plates was lethal when inhaled or absorbed through the skin. The author discusses the moral, symbolic, and legal implications of this firt recorded instance of corporate officials in America being charged with murder for the work-related death of an employee.

5 / The Invisible Risk . . .

MARK REUTTER

"Think before you act. *Your Safety Is In Your Hands.*" These words are stenciled onto the door of a mechanic's shanty tucked underneath a railroad trestle at Sparrows Point, Maryland.

The shanty—windowless, scattered with tools—was the early morning refuge of Earl Barley. About an hour before the start of the daylight shift, he would push open the rusty metal door, sit down at the center table and begin a routine honed by 23 years of work at the huge Bethlehem Steel Corporation mill near Baltimore. He made tea with hot water from his Thermos, had a smoke and, as a radio played in the background, changed into his work clothes.

On January 27, 1979, Barley was assigned as usual to a blast furnace repair gang. The other men in the gang knew his habits well. They knew he would leave the shanty at seven o'clock and walk up an adjoining narrow alley to meet them.

When he did not appear by 7:15, one of the men started down the alley to find him. Although his view was obscured by steam, Paul Ruszin saw something on the ground. He picked up his pace, then broke into a run. Outside the shanty door, face down, lay Earl Barley, half-dressed and with one shoe on.

Suspecting a heart attack, Ruszin went for help and came back with several other workers. A minute or two later, as an ambulance attendant rushed to Barley, Ruszin started to wobble. He lurched backward and, like a drunken marionette, threw a stilted punch toward Charlie Shears. *What the hell is going on?* Shears wondered. *Two men aren't going to get heart attacks like this, are they?*

Shears surveyed the maze of pipes and exhaust stacks that climbed a hundred feet above the alley. Nothing unusual. He sniffed. Pretty much the normal smell of the furnaces. More men gathered. Shears looked around the dark alley and caught sight of a cat—a large, gray cat. The cat was dead. "This man didn't have any heart attack. He was gassed," Shears shouted, then blacked out.

Unknown to the workers, or to anyone else at the plant, gas from a major blast furnace pipeline was escaping into the alley. The gas—

colorless, tasteless and virtually odorless—contained a concentration of carbon monoxide so potent it would produce bizarre effects within minutes: hallucinations, convulsions, loss of memory. In a few more minutes, unconsciousness would set in, then death from asphyxiation. The leak that morning killed Earl Barley. Ruszin and five other men recovered after receiving emergency treatment in an oxygen pressure chamber. Fifteen additional workers, including Shears, were examined for less severe carbon monoxide poisoning.

Afterward, officials from Bethlehem Steel declined to discuss the accident with reporters except to say that its cause was "a mystery." A spokesperson emphasized that steel making was dangerous work which requires employees to be ever vigilant of their safety—just as the company's slogans warn. As the TV news crews filmed, one official read a statement saying, "Concern for employee safety is paramount at Sparrow's Point."

No one asked questions about the similarity between this accident and a string of other fatalities and injuries at the steel plant. But the accidents fit a common pattern, one that George Bourne, Joey Rothenberg, Walter Coonts and Midge Hall knew well.

In numerous cases, management neglected to take elementary safety precautions, failed to maintain hazardous equipment and ignored patently dangerous conditions. This disregard for the welfare of workers is not confined to Bethlehem Steel. Throughout the industry—in the Pittsburgh Steel Belt; in Gary, Indiana; along the East Chicago waterfront, and on Ohio's Mahoning River—serious injuries have been on the upswing as mill superintendents try to find new ways to speed up aging machinery and boost production. Yet the high injury rate, like the carbon monoxide that killed Earl Barley, is a problem that is largely invisible to the world outside of steel manufacturing.

Life at "The Point"

Covering four square miles of former marshland at the mouth of Baltimore Harbor, Sparrows Point is the largest steel works on the East Coast and the third-largest in the country. There are more than 1,500 buildings and furnaces. Several are as high as the nearby skyscrapers of Baltimore; others extend a third of a mile in length and are three city blocks wide. Flanking these buildings—eclipsed by their soaring verticals and broad horizontals—are hundreds of structures big in their own right: cylindrical stoves rising 12 stories and girdled by pipe; coke ovens, 635 of them, resembling monstrous auto batteries; pitch-roofed stockhouses and oblong engine rooms; cranes perched on towers or cantilevered across truss bridges; elevators; conveyors; storage tanks; railroad trestles.

Each structure contributes to the making and molding of steel. Furnaces produce up to 800 tons of steel an hour in gargantuan ladles heated to 2,900 degrees Fahrenheit. The sparkling orange steel is hauled to finishing mills, where powerful rolling machines flatten, squeeze, pound, twist, shape, chemically and electrically treat, slice, spin and smooth the metal into hundreds of products that are essential to American industry.

Auto plants in the Northeast depend on steel sheets rolled in the hot-strip mills. Tinplate is sold to toy, can, bottle cap and Venetian blind manufacturers. Bridges, boilers and office buildings across the country are held together with steel plates and beams from Sparrows Point. Every year the plant's wire mill chops up 100,000 miles of steel wire to make three billion nails.

Like most major steel centers, Sparrows Point is a city unto itself. A 165-member company policy force, given full law enforcement powers by the state of Maryland, patrols the grounds. The company has its own fire department, railroad and hospital-dispensary. Although the company town no longer exists, many of its traditions remain. A spacious country club continues to serve as a protective cocoon for management; and black workers, in numbers beyond what should be expected, still wind up on coke oven teams, on bull gangs and in other hot, dirty jobs.

Twenty thousand people work at "The Point." When the shift changes, cars and vans by the hundreds flow from the company parking lots—big American-made ones: Impalas and LTDs, aging Cadillacs, Mustangs with chrome-capped racing tires, Malibus and Thunderbirds, rainbow-colored Chevy vans on jacked-up chassis. They gun up Seventh Street to Bethlehem Boulevard or wind along Tin Mill Road. Within moments, they become thin pencil marks against the huge sweeps of steel, brick and smoke.

Sparrows Point was the crowning achievement of Charles M. Schwab, an entrepreneur of enormous ambition. The mill was established in 1887 but grew slowly until Schwab came to Baltimore in 1916. A protégé of Andrew Carnegie's, Schwab helped Carnegie and J. P. Morgan form the biggest trust in the world—the U.S. Steel Corporation—then left its presidency in 1902 to take over a small business in northern Pennsylvania.

Within a decade he had transformed the Bethlehem Steel Corporation into the second-largest steel-producer (after U.S. Steel) and the nation's preeminent munitions manufacturer, "equipped to turn out every instrument of warfare used on land or sea," in the words of a New York newspaper.

Money was the great motivator for Schwab—he spent it ardently, using it to build, among other structures, the most lavish private residence in Manhattan—and money was the key to his management system. When he took over Bethlehem, he introduced a bonus plan that directly rewarded or punished an employee on the basis of daily output. If a worker was unable to reach a predetermined tonnage level, he faced dismissal or demotion to a less demanding job. If he succeeded the figure, he received a bonus—and so did his foreman and other supervisors. Since base pay determined bonus pay, a hard-working employee received rather small increments. But incentive pay could double the salary of a mill superintendent. And in a good year the top executives at Bethlehem made out handsomely, each receiving incentive bonuses that ranged between $100,000 and $1 million.

With the opening of the Panama Canal in 1914, Schwab foresaw the economic advantages of a tidewater steel mill. Rich iron-ore deposits in South America could be shipped cheaply to Sparrows Point, and finished products could be sent through the canal to the steel-hungry West Coast. After purchasing the complex in 1916, Schwab announced that Bethlehem would pour $50 million into plant improvements. He called the commitment the largest single investment ever made by an American company.

During the next 40 years the mill grew relentlessly, becoming the pace-setter of the steel industry. By 1957, it was the largest steel-producer in the world, employing about 30,000 hourly workers. But as steel industry profits dipped in the 1960s and new Soviet and Japanese mills outstripped American efficiency, expansion halted and the work force was pared down. In 1971, steel output was cut back and several thousand employees were laid off.

The Fatal Output

Accidents have always been a fact of life at Sparrows Point. Until recently, though, they did not have to be reported to the government, and Bethlehem never volunteered the information. "If a man got killed or badly hurt, often people never heard of it," remembers a 74-year-old woman who spent her life at Sparrows Point and worked in the tin mill.

In the old days, she said, the coffin and mourning party were transported to a graveyard in the city aboard a specially designed streetcar named Dolores. In 1918, she and her family took Dolores to a Catholic cemetery in West Baltimore. They were burying her brother, a water boy who had died of lockjaw after his leg was mangled in a mill accident. He was 14.

Last year, 5,304 accident-related injuries were reported among the 17,500 blue-collar workers at the plant, or one injury for every 3.3 workers. About one-quarter of the accidents were serious enough to require an employee to temporarily transfer to another job or stay out of work altogether. The 649 workers who could not work needed a long time to recuperate—a month each on the average.

This high injury rate is typical of steel manufacturing throughout the country. Steel making is dangerous work, as hazardous as coal mining or building construction, according to statistics compiled by OSHA, the Occupational Safety and Health Administration. Some OSHA officials believe the accident toll in these industries is even higher than figures indicate. Certain injuries, they say, go unreported because federal regulations largely leave it up to management to determine what constitutes a so-called recordable injury.

OSHA regulations do not require employers to divulge detailed accident data, but Bethlehem tabulates such statistics for an in-house newsletter to supervisors at Sparrows Point. These reports show that major accidents in 1978, for example, caused the following: six deaths (each occurring in a separate incident), one coma, seven amputations, 70 eye injuries, 86 back injuries and hernias, 181 burns, 205 fractures and dislocations, and 395 large cuts and puncture wounds. (There were six more deaths last year. Three men were killed at the steel mill; three others died from accidents which occurred at the shipbuilding yard.)

The company also compiles injury figures by the month. In 1978, the monthly total hovered around 350 during the winter, rose to 500 in the summer and dropped below 400 by November. Plotted on a bar graph, the monthly injury rate has a similar contour to another graph that appears monthly in the supervisors' newsletter—the graph of steel production at Sparrows Point.

A Clear Violation?

Earl Barley's death from carbon monoxide poisoning shook up George Bourne. They were buddies, men who worked out of the same shop in the same craft. As millwrights, they repaired blast furnaces and related equipment. Working in hot, claustrophobic areas, often unable to speak over the shattering noise, the men had to depend on each other's reflexes and intuition. Bourne shared another bond with Barley. They were both raised in the mountains, Bourne in eastern Tennessee and Barley in western Maryland, and Bourne knew the code of the hills when a buddy's honor was at stake. "From where I was born," he explained one day, "you don't back down, and I got scars to prove it."

Bourne did not believe that Barley was the victim of a freak accident. He had seen too much the previous year, when he served as chairman of a union committee that investigated accidents in one section of the mill. In March 1978, a worker drowned after a truck he was driving slid into a waste-water pond. Then two veteran workers collapsed from heat stroke on the same day—one later died and the other suffered severe and permanent brain damage. Then a hot-blastman was killed at C Furnace. Then a pit worker at No. 4 open-hearth. Four fatalities in ten months—the biggest toll in more than a decade in the steel-making part of the plant. And there were two more deaths in the finishing mills.

In each case Bourne's committee found—and Maryland safety and health inspectors later confirmed—that the accidents could have been avoided if Bethlehem had taken basic safety precautions. In two of the cases, the victims might have survived if the company had had better rescue methods.

While investigating the Barley accident, Bourne was particularly haunted by the death of Robert Carter three months earlier. Carter, training to be a hot-blastman, was found unconscious less than 200 feet from where Barley later collapsed. Both men died of carbon monoxide poisoning. The gas escaped in both cases from a dilapidated furnace system that had been scheduled to be shut down in 1977 but was kept in operation to save money.

In each incident there was no equipment in the area that could detect carbon monoxide leaks. Nor was there an alarm system to warn employees of danger or gas masks to protect them from the fumes. When the colorless, tasteless and virtually odorless gas seeped from a pipe, it was up to the employee to recognize the hazard and get out of the area quickly.

In the Carter case, the company committed such flagrant violations of safety standards that a $24,000 fine was levied against it by the Maryland Occupational Safety and Health Agency. A week before his death, Carter was exposed to a heavy dose of carbon monoxide at the furnace. He was treated at the company dispensary but was not informed of the cause of his illness. Although company officials knew that Carter had been subjected to dangerous levels of the gas, they took no steps to stop the leakage, state officials charged.

Barley was killed when a pressurized water seal blew at the rear of the furnace, releasing gas from a pipeline into the shack where he was dressing. Enraged by the accident, George Bourne used his self-obtained knowledge of the pipeline system to try to figure out what had happened. He knew that the company, in an effort to cut costs, had been trying to increase gas pressure throughout the system. Under Bourne's questioning, a Bethlehem official conceded that the company did not really know what effect these pressure changes might have on the pipeline. More resilient water seals were being installed, but the company had not gotten around to replacing the seal which later failed, causing Earl Barley's death.

Bourne presented this and other evidence to state safety inspectors, but they told him that the information did not show a clear violation of a safety standard. The inspectors added that they did not possess enough expertise to question Bethlehem's assertion that the seal should not have blown.

Bourne was stymied. As weeks turned into months and no violation notice was issued, he became increasingly bitter. One morning he vented his frustration inside the union hall, "Barley was the type of person who was very conscious about gas," he said. "I think he knew he was gettin' gassed, but the man didn't have a chance. You can't smell the gas until there's a lot of it. It has a musty, moldy smell. And by then," he said, knocking his right hand on the table for emphasis, "that gas is so damn concentrated that a couple of whiffs and you're gone."

Thickly built, with a robust beard and curly black hair wreathing his face, Bourne gives the impression of being fearless. But carbon monoxide is an enemy that cannot be seen. Even an experienced man has trouble detecting that musty odor in an already smelly environment. Bourne, who barely escaped from a gas leak once, remembers what rushed through his mind: "I'm in a tunnel, in a hole, and I'm looking out and I'm fading back real slow."

A Compensable Case

Joey Rothenberg was sitting in a wheelchair at the Sparrows Point dispensary, in terrible pain, when her foreman told her to look at the bright side.

"He came over and said, 'At least now you can work daylight through the Christmas holiday.' I said, 'What?' 'You know, you can come in and sit around the office, and if you feel like it you can help with the paperwork.' "

The 28-year-old crane operator, whose mouth had just been smashed in an accident, begged off. But the offers kept coming. Twice in the next two days a higher-ranking foreman called her at home. "He was very friendly, the big father-figure, and he said, 'I hate to see you hurting before the holidays. Why don't you come in the office and help us with the paperwork? If you want to, you can sleep.' " Not only did the supervisor offer to drive her to work, Rothenberg said, "He told me he could give me a better pay rate."

Instead of going to work she went to a doctor, and he ordered her to stay home. After that the calls stopped. Rothenberg said she was not surprised. She had become a "compensable" case; that is, 72 hours had lapsed and the company had to report her injury to the workmen's compensation board.

She was off work for three weeks, nursing a shattered front tooth, stitched-up lip and bruised hand. She had time to contemplate the irony that the foreman who tried to avoid reporting her accident could have prevented it.

Rothenberg was assigned to operate a crane that had been in mothballs for eight years, but which was needed to handle an increase in orders. The crane constantly broke down and had no emergency brake.

On the night of December 12, 1978, Rothenberg was having trouble with the crane's lifting "dog" but was told to continue working. As the crane neared the end of its tracks, the motor suddenly cut off, automatically shutting down the breaking system. Without emergency brakes, the 25-ton crane glided forward and slammed against the rail stops, flinging Rothenberg against the cab window. She was helped down to an ambulance station where she began to hallucinate. "I kept thinking I was back in that cab, lying there on the floor."

After being treated at the dispensary, she was placed in a wheelchair. It was then that her foreman came in to make his offer. About the same time, electricians began working on the crane. They were putting in an emergency brake "on orders from above," a member of the crew told her later.

The Human Element

The day after Joey Rothenberg's accident, the general manager of Sparrows Point, Russell R. Jones, discussed the relationship between profits and maintenance at the plant. He spoke at an engineers club meeting at the company's private country club near the steel mill.

"Both maintenance forces and costs must follow operational levels," he said. "In other words, when we are in periods of high production and we are making money, we can spend it. The converse is also true. When production levels are down and we are not making money, we cannot spend it." He allowed that "obviously this is not the best situation for maintenance," but to do otherwise would be "contrary to financial reality."

Jones did not discuss the relationship between maintenance and safety. Instead, he called the plant's safety record excellent and attributed the rise in injuries to "extenuating circumstances."

His speech came at a time when accidents had claimed the most lives in a year since 1962. The injury toll was the highest since 1974, when the mill had had several thousand more employees. In five of the six fatalities in 1978, state safety officials had charged that Bethlehem had committed "serious" or "willful" violations of safety laws and had fined the company a total of $62,800. Another $10,400 was assessed against the company for exposing coke-oven workers to excessive amounts of coal tars and benzene, two cancer-causing substances.

Jones, a husky, distinguished-looking man in his mid-50s, would not talk to the press about the accidents or fines. But, speaking from the podium at the Sparrows Point Country Club, he made it clear to his subordinates that Bethlehem would not stray from the economic course it had charted since the late 1960s.

That course meant that high-speed machinery went without routine repair until it broke down and had to be fixed. Jobs not directly tied to production were eliminated or combined with other jobs. After several poor years, company profits surged to $225 million in 1978. Although respectable, the profit margin was "still short of our goal," Lewis W. Foy, chairman of Bethlehem, told stockholders, adding that his objective for 1979 and 1980 was to "move further toward the goal of attaining rates of return at least equal to the average returns of all manufacturing companies."

Is there a connection between this so-called productivity drive and the number of accidents at Sparrows Point? Of course not, Chairman Foy told the *Baltimore Sun;* he conceded later that the rate of serious accidents had risen at most of the company's plants.

In the interview, he did not lament the workers' injuries but called the accidents "a tragedy from the standpoint of our safety record." Employing artfully vague prose, Foy made it appear that management accepted responsibility for workplace safety while simultaneously implying that workers were exclusively to blame for accidents. His was a variant of the old argument that malingering workers cause machines to malfunction. Or as he put it, "We are taking every measure we can possibly think of to increase the intensity of our safety program. . . . We are inspecting all of our equipment and machinery down there to make sure that it is safe from every human element."

For ten years Walter Coonts watched "human elements" get hurt on the machines that make heavy-duty wire at The Point. In 1973, he thought he was in a position to do something about it.

Appointed secretary of a union safety committee, Coonts began to document the hazards of the 85 wire machines. He knew them well; in the early 1960s he had trained on the machines and said that "they were so dangerous I wouldn't work the job." The danger stemmed from the absence of shields over the rotating disks, which pulled wire through cutting dies at speeds up to 1,500 feet per minute.

Shortly after Coonts joined the union committee, there was another bad accident. A worker's hand, caught in the rushing wire, was mutilated in an unguarded "ripper block." Several of the employee's fingers had to be amputated. Coonts wrote the first of several memos to the company safety department urging the placement of shields "so employees are out of reach and danger of all moving parts."

Nothing was done. He argued repeatedly for the shields at the monthly labor-management safety meetings. Finally, in August 1974, company officials told Coonts, the minutes of the meeting show, that "supervision is presently developing plans" to install the guards.

"But 1975 dawned and only *one* machine of the 85 was shielded. Several meetings with management produced more vague assurances. Then the "front office" vetoed the project, Coonts was told. With production levels down, the company said it could not afford the $80,000 price tag.

Even before this rebuff, Coonts said the committee work was wearing him down. Day after day he dealt with foremen—some sympathetic to safety, others indifferent—who were rewarded only according to their tonnage figures. He haggled with safety department officials who admitted that they were just filling a position. He talked with employees who were worried about working conditions and employees who invoked the issue of safety to settle a grudge with a supervisor. But thanks to Bethlehem's incentive system, it's the person who works quickly—not necessarily safely—who makes the money.

"Sure, some guys take short cuts. The foreman looks the other way; he wants 'em to," Coonts explained, sitting in the living room of his ranch house. "There's pressure on you all the time, from the company and from yourself. It's always keep up, keep up, got to catch up."

Coonts left the safety committee in mid-1975. He continued to work in the wire department, usually within earshot of the *ratatat* beat of steel wire being drawn into carbide dies.

Death on the Wire

On June 16, 1978, at 11:15 a.m., 29-year-old Robert E. Hall was pulled into a wire machine. He died instantly. There were no reported eyewitnesses. Investigators reconstructed the following events: Hall was working on No. 8 bull-block when his gloved left hand became entwined in the running wire. He was swept off his feet and flung headfirst into an unshielded metal spool. Halfway around the spool, his body set off an emergency switch, and the machine stopped.

Early that afternoon, two officials from Bethlehem notified Midge Hall of the accident. They provided few details. Seven months pregnant with her fourth child, she was comforted by her sister while Hall's father and brother Frank rushed down to the wire department. Frank almost got into a fight when a company official said the accident was caused by "operator error."

After an investigation, the Maryland Occupational Safety and Health Agency fined Bethlehem $27,200 for "serious" safety violations. Each violation involved the absence of shields around the wire machines. If the No. 8 bull-block had been shielded, Hall would not have been pulled into the machine and killed, the agency's chief inspector reported.

In late August, Midge Hall gave birth to Stephen, a healthy seven-pounder. Several days later a newspaper article disclosed that the Maryland safety agency had *withdrawn* a violation notice the previous year that would have required Bethlehem to place shields around the wire machines. The notice and a $150 fine were dropped after company executives protested the notice at a private meeting with safety agency officials.

After reading the newspaper article, Midge Hall said she became very upset. Her in-laws and neighbors urged her to sue Bethlehem Steel. She hired a lawyer suggested by a friend; but after researching the state law, he reported back that a suit would be folly. Like most states, Maryland requires a plaintiff to prove that a company "willfully and deliberately" intended to injure an employee. To establish gross negligence or violation of safety laws was not enough, he said, adding that a suit could jeopardize the money she would receive under workmen's compensation.

How could a law be written like that? she wondered. *How could a judge "let them get away with it?"* Midge Hall talked, and still talks, about a suit. The money doesn't matter: "I want them to know he wasn't just a number."

Midge Joseph met Bob Hall in 1970. She was down from Cumberland, Maryland, visiting her sister, and Bob came over. "I guess that was it." She was 19 and they were married within the year. A photograph shows both with radiant smiles. Midge was the shorter of the two, with a round face and large dark eyes. Bob had curly dirty-blond hair and was thin. He came from a family of steelworkers. His father, mother and two older brothers all had worked at The Point. Shortly before he met Midge, he too joined Bethlehem Steel.

They saved, made it through a long layoff and in 1976 bought a two-story brick rowhouse in Middle River, ten miles north of the plant. Bob was a quiet man who spent his spare time repairing and riding motorcycles, according to Midge. Early in 1978 he decided to transfer from the blast furnace to the wire department.

"He wanted to spend more time at home with the kids, and he thought it was a cleaner and safer job," Midge says. "He saw a lot over there [at the furnaces]. Just before he left, he saw a guy step into a bucket of whatever it was and it burned his boot right off his foot. . . . He didn't want to go through another summer there. When it's 100 degrees outside and you're going into the furnace area, it's gotta be pure hell in there for those men. He'd come home black as the ace of spades and go right to sleep."

The children occupy Midge Hall's life now. "They're pretty good, but I lose my temper very easily. I realize it's all on me. I'm full boss." Eight-year-old Lori talks about her father but doesn't weep. Tara Lynn, age six, prods her mother to buy her another daddy, and Bobby, who recently turned five, still goes through crying spells. "He tells me he's my man," Midge says, holding two-year-old Stephen, who has his father's blond hair and angular face.

On a bad night, when Midge retreats to the downstairs couch, her thoughts go back to the place where her husband worked for eight years. Since that day, when the company officials came to her door with the news that her husband was dead, she has heard nothing from Bethlehem Steel.

Walter Coonts did not know Bob Hall and did not hear of his death until the day after it happened. "It kind of stunned me. You know, I had that feeling it was going to happen all along and finally it happened." Coonts' soft mountain twang is drawn out, hard to hear. He shakes his head.

What effect has the accident had on safety? "Well, it's put them over a barrel, that's what it's done," Coonts said recently. "Of course, they say they're sorry and they hope it don't ever happen again and that they're going to do everything they can to prevent it. But I don't think their attitude has ever changed."

Why? Coonts' blue eyes flicker. He lets out a chuckle before explaining. Accidents will continue, he maintains, because it is cheaper for Bethlehem to pay safety fines and workmen's compensation than to fix its machinery and change its production system. His reasoning, expressed by many other steelworkers, has long been discounted by safety professionals. But with accident rates showing few signs of significantly receding, some prominent officials are now echoing these sentiments.

Safety does not necessarily pay, Ray Marshall, secretary of the U.S. Labor Department, told a Senate committee last year. The low cost of workmen's compensation benefits—less than 1.5 percent of the average employer's payroll—"provides few economic incentives," Marshall said, especially when this cost can be absorbed in the price of a product. Moreover, fines by OSHA or state safety agencies rarely exceed $10,000 for a fatal accident. Such fines are negligible to giants such as Bethlehem and U.S. Steel, whose individual plants often boast payrolls in excess of $500,000 a day.

Nine years after the passage of the OSHA Act, the agency has promulgated numerous regulations but has done little to force the industry to alter the practices and pressures—the noise and dust, the speedups and equipment breakdowns—that lead to accidents.

After accidents claimed another two lives at Sparrows Point last year, the union newspaper made a modest proposal. It recommended that general manager Russell Jones leave his office at quitting time and go over to the clockhouses. There, the paper said, he could personally "congratulate employees for making it through another day at the steel mills."

6 / Death by Cotton Dust

RICHARD GUARASCI
St. Lawrence University

WORKING FOR West Point-Pepperell Company will kill Nat Wilkins.*
Slowly but surely, they took his labor, and they are taking his life too.
Nat Wilkins can't breath. He suffers from the continuing strangulation of brown lung disease (byssinosis). He entrusted his working life
to the owners and managers of the mill valley surrounding Opelika,
Alabama. He quietly exchanged hard work in dirty and noisy conditions for a steady but poorly paid job. Nat Wilkins lived his life on
trust—in God, country, and the mill. In the end, the mill will fail him.
And worse, those responsible could have prevented it all along.
Textile corporations, their insurance companies and company doctors, local officials and politicians, all of them could easily have saved
the lives of the many Nat Wilkins who litter the textile industry with a
legacy of preventable occupational disease and human suffering. Nat
Wilkins received some compensation only because he brought a class
action suit against the managers of the Alabama plant on behalf of all
brown lung victims. Because of the tireless dedication of the Southern
Poverty Law Center in Montgomery, Nat won a generous out-of-
court settlement. More important, one of the depositions taken
proved to be a "smoking gun," indicting the entire cotton textile
industry and its allies in what can only be termed a "corporate cover-
up." For years, the industry denied knowledge of the lethal effects of
cotton dust on its workers. It did not acknowledge employee health
problems until the 1970s. In the Wilkins case, damaging testimony
was given by a medical investigator for Liberty Mutual, the leading
workman's compensation insurer for the textile industry. Dr. Joseph
Bosworth, retired "loss-prevention investigator" for Liberty Mutual,
recognized as early as the 1950s that many textile workers had brown
lung. In the chambers of a Florida law office, after being subpoenaed,

---

*The persons cited in the case studies discussed in this chapter were
interviewed by the author.

Dr. Bosworth testified to corporate negligence in ignoring, if not actually hiding, knowledge of brown lung among workers. Wilkins's attorney read to Bosworth from a transcript of a recorded phone conversation between one of the investigators and himself. They pressed Bosworth to confirm, in his deposition, what he had said in his phone conversation—that textile companies knew, in the 1950s, of brown lung disease among its employees, and instead of informing and protecting their workers, these companies "ran from it . . . because it threatened them with a wholesale cost." The following excerpt is from Bosworth's testimony.[1]

Q. Okay Dr. Bosworth, what did you mean when you said, "This is one of the things that cramps the style of medicine and occupational medicine, is the legal side of the people that paid"?

A. Employers notoriously have been charged with doing a lot to employees that maybe they did in some places, maybe they didn't, and they are leery about starting wholesale information of reminding them, "Now, look, you ought to sue me for this."

Q. As far as you know, Dr. Bosworth, employers aren't anxious to have workers' compensation claims filed against them?

A. Certainly not. They're human.

Q. It says [in a transcript of a recorded phone conversation],
"Rick: . . . was that standard procedure with Liberty Mutual or was that something that the mills required?"
"Doctor: Well Liberty Mutual couldn't violate the wishes of the mills because they were insuring them."
Now is that statement you made true or false?

A. That statement is true.

Q. "Rick: I see and that . . . Did you ever determine what percentage of workers . . ."
"Doctor (Bosworth): No and we didn't look for percentages. We were not looking for that. We were running from it, really."
"Rick: Running from it?"
"Doctor: That's right."
"Rick: What? I don't understand."
"Doctor: Well, we didn't want any more claims. The clients [textile mills] didn't want anymore claims on 'em then they had to have."
Were the statements that you made there that I just read, Dr. Bosworth, true or false?

A. They're true in certain lights. I would have answered it differently, had I known the man who was asking the questions, what he was.

Q. Now turn to page four, please.
"Doctor: and the industries, when they found out about it, of course, they were scared to death. They didn't know what was

going to happen, because they could have been a wholesale cost to 'em, and they didn't want any part of it."
Now was that statement true or false?

A.   The statement was true. You wouldn't either.

"You wouldn't either," want any part of compensation claims for the gradual strangulation by cotton dust, unless, of course you worked in the mills.

Cotton Dust and the Textile Legacy

The textile industry, located in small company-owned mill towns throughout the southeastern United States, dates back to the Reconstruction period following the Civil War, although there are histories of mills in operation in the Carolinas as early as the Jacksonian period. Until the recent advances of the civil rights movement, it was an industry for low-income white workers plucked from the failing farms of the South to provide them with an advantage over their black neighbors. In the spirit of such oppressive systems, all collective efforts were viewed (correctly so) as threats to the status quo. But no activities were so violently opposed as workers' attempts to unionize.

The beauty of the Carolinas, the heart of the textile manufacturing industry, is scarred by the sight of its textile workers, bent from shortness of breath, prematurely disabled by the suffocating grip of cotton dust they unnecessarily inhaled in their daily labor. In the struggle for corporate growth and profits, the lungs of these workers have been mortgaged to the chronic, painful sickness—"brown lung." After working all their adult lives, sometimes from childhood, many cotton textile workers have found themselves permanently disabled at about fifty years of age, hard pressed to sleep or breathe, faced with a desperate but most likely unsuccessful struggle for disability income from workmen's compensation. Many share the feelings of Paul Cline, a South Carolina textile worker for over forty years. "The good Lord gives man the breath to breathe and I don't think the textile mills have the right to take it away. They sacrifice our lives for profits."

There are just under 400,000 textile workers in the Carolinas and approximately 115,000 of them are exposed to cotton dust. It is estimated that between 18,000 and 35,000 Carolinians suffer from byssinosis, but in the history of both the North and South Carolina Industrial Commissions (workmen's compensation boards) until 1980 only 320 disability awards for brown lung were granted. The average award in North Carolina has been $13,000; in South Carolina $14,000. These grand sums are supposed to provide for the estimated remaining years of the recipient's life in lieu of employment. Sometimes, the money must be used to pay medical bills. Many of the "lucky" 320 who were certified "disabled" from byssinosis could have, if healthy, worked many more years until retirement. The dangers of contracting byssinosis are kept from the employees by the mill owners. Furthermore, state agencies and departments of labor have failed to inspect, with any degree of consistency or thoroughness, the hazardous conditions of the mills. Regulatory agencies have written numerous and unwarranted extensions for compliance into their reports.[2]

Stranglehold of Power

The history of compensation in the Carolinas is one of corporate power, governmental complicity, and worker ignorance. While only two percent of all other compensation cases are contested by employers in the Carolinas, until 1980, eighty percent of the North Carolina and one hundred percent of the South Carolina brown lung cases were litigated by the textile companies. Since then, worker insurgencies have softened company resistance only modestly. Both industrial commissions have resisted byssinosis disability claims even though the disease has been recognized since the late eighteenth century, and has been a compensable disease in Britain since World War II.

The "compensation-safety apparatus" of the Carolinas has proven totally ineffective in forcing the textile companies to absorb the environmental and medical costs of byssinosis; it has in fact coupled company neglect with tacit government sanction. For example, between 1974 and 1980, 101 of the 128 mills that had been inspected in South Carolina exceeded permissible dust limits. One company, Hermitage Mills, which has fought its citations in the state courts, took more than five years to correct documented violations. In North Carolina, 128 of 210 mills inspected were cited for dust violations, and in 75 percent of these, dust levels three times the permissible standard were found. The average time allowed for compliance was twenty months, but some companies took three years to achieve compliance. The average penalty levied by both Carolinas' Occupational Safety and Health Administrations is approximately $50. By early 1980, neither had ever taken an employer to court for failure to pay their fines, and South Carolina had collected only 44 percent of its fines for 1979. Since 1981, OSHA has imposed a stronger cotton dust standard, improving the record slightly, but major enforcement problems remain.

The pernicious occupational conditions and governmental policies that permit byssinosis to debilitate possibly as many as 35,000 Carolinians is founded on authoritarian, and often, illegal rule in the workplace. J. P. Stevens, the second largest textile manufacturer to Burlington Mills (Stevens' sales were $2.4 billion in 1979.), has been characterized by the National Labor Relations Board (NLRB) as the greatest labor-law violator in the nation. It has been cited twenty-two times for illegal labor practices, many involving firing or disciplining workers who have complained or organized for a safe and healthy workplace.[3] The prevalence of disabling working conditions in the textile industry depends on a foundation of managerial domination and governmental sanction.

Roanoke Rapids, North Carolina

Examples of corporate negligence are all too apparent in Roanoke Rapids. In 1974, workers at the J. P. Stevens Textile Mills voted to join the Amalgamated Clothing and Textile Workers Union (ACTWU). Although the local won a negotiated contract, the conflict between Stevens and ACTWU has taken on the characteristics of a tense chess game that will significantly affect numerous other ACTWU attempts to unionize Stevens throughout the South. Stevens demands impossible concessions, hoping to goad the union into a strike so that management will be able to shift production to its more than eighty plants elsewhere in the South. The union seeks contracts that will demonstrate real gains to workers at the other plants.

Against the backdrop of this industrial drama, the town of Roanoke Rapids houses many textile workers, old before their time and ill from brown lung after years of working at Stevens. The work histories of former employees attest to industrial negligence, authoritarian rule in the workplace, and pernicious administration of government regulations.

Homes in Roanoke Rapids range from converted mill houses and one-family homes to more modest structures, dilapidated from lack of care by displaced farmers and the unemployed. This calm and peaceful veneer provides a jarring contrast to the testimony heard at the local office of the Brown Lung Association. Descriptions of company practices range from tragic negligence to callous domination; my encounters with numerous textile workers confirm these descriptions.

Percy Sutton worked for forty-two years in the mills. He receives no pension and, although he suffers from the progressive breathlessness of byssinosis, he receives no compensation. He is a deeply religious fundamentalist who trusts in the Lord to see him through hardship, but the realization that years of underpaid labor have brought him a shortened life and an expensive illness have led him to participate in a collective action to redress the injustice of the "textile system." In describing the condition of the mills, he says, "You could see the dust . . . we had no protective equipment. They put in air conditioning [in his last years of work] and they bricked up the walls. I could take the cotton out of my mouth after work."

A heavy set, elderly man in his 70s, James Tripp began working in the Roanoke Rapids mills in 1940. He served in World War II, seeing action. Now he sits in a chair, able to sleep only a few hours at a time because of his breathing problems. He takes pills constantly to alleviate his condition, but they only reduce his congestion for a few hours. James is quiet and he rarely volunteers any information. Only after some inquiries does he disclose his true age, which he believes to be in the late 40s. In addition to the physical burden of his disease, James is emotionally paralyzed by having to decide either to pursue a workmen's compensation award from the North Carolina Industrial Commission, or to settle with J. P. Stevens for significantly less. Since brown lung is virtually impossible to diagnose from symptoms alone, the lengthy compensation-hearing process will probably take over two years and will require James to testify and retestify, to be examined and cross-examined by lawyers of Stevens and Liberty Mutual, Steven's insurance carrier. An important part of the questioning will concern James's recollection of working conditions during his more than thirty years in the mills, as well as his personal health habits, particularly smoking. James fears that he will inadvertently confuse his facts and cause the Industrial Commission to rule against him on the grounds of his credibility. Even though James Tripp obviously deserves a full award, the fear of losing all compensation because of his own illiteracy or tension overwhelms him. James Tripp, a war veteran, is a proud person who has made himself a life by dint of his labor and courage. It's that courage that byssinosis wears down.

John Henry Moore, another disabled textile worker, was denied compensation by the Industrial Commission because his credibility was questioned. After thirty-nine years of dust-filled work in the opening room where he quickly opened bags of raw cotton to feed sorting machines, John Henry Moore failed at his first attempt to receive brown lung compensation. Even though breathing tests and medical evidence clearly suggested byssinosis, a doctor for the Industrial Commission questioned whether John Henry was really a brown lung victim. Mr. Moore told me, "He got hot with me because I couldn't read and write . . . I never learned because when my daddy said plow the mule, I plowed the mule. I had not time to learn readin' and writin.' I can't read nor write but I did work for thirty-nine years. Even some people with good sense can't work thirty-nine years. I had sense enough to work."

After John Henry Moore's case received public attention in the Carolina press, the Industrial Commission agreed to re-open it. The interviewing physician in the initial medical diagnosis was Dr. Mario Battigelli. He never asked Moore about the classic symptoms of byssinosis, therefore Moore didn't volunteer such information. On that basis, Dr. Battigelli decided the patient was not suffering from brown lung. He was denied compensation because compensation law does not require "presumptive diagosis" as it does under special federal legislation for black lung victims of the coal miners.[4] Six months after Battigelli examined Moore, Dr. Herbert Seiker, a Duke University lung specialist, diagnosed byssinosis.

All too often, the local doctors in mill towns are in the employ of the textile companies, who until recently, denied that byssinosis existed, even though the trade journal, Textile World, published an article about the disease as early as 1940. In fact, ten of twelve doctors on the North Carolina Textile Occupational Disease Panel are employed by textile companies—Cannon, Fieldcrest, Cone, Burlington, and J. P. Stevens among others. The nexus of textile companies, health professionals, insurance companies, and governmental officials was an insurmountable obstacle for disabled workers before the existence of the Brown Lung Association (BLA).

The BLA office in Roanoke Rapids is filled with an endless parade of byssinosis sufferers, all with lengthy work experience but few with pensions from J. P. Stevens. Some had been given compensation settlements, others had filed and were involved in the lengthy and stressful hearing process. Their descriptions of working conditions in Roanoke Rapids can be compared with Charles Dickens's graphic descriptions of industrial England.

The case of Bud and Louise Harrison, both millworkers, captures other aspects of the brown lung victim's plight. Both Bud and Louise began working in the mills when they reached adolescence. She was thirteen years old and living on a farm when a mill supervisor was sent around to rural areas to "hunt up" some cheap labor. He visited her farm and hired the entire family as one working unit, including her father and his four girls. All of them worked twelve to sixteen hours a day, six days a week, at the end of which they were given one paycheck. They lived in company-owned housing and shopped in company-owned stores. Bud began working in the mill when he was about fifteen years old. They married shortly after.

Bud served in World War II with distinction and was decorated for bravery in combat. For a time, he returned to the mills, but with the help of the GI Bill, he attended trade school in Chicago and later worked in the Virginia shipyards where he was consistently exposed to asbestos. Bud returned to the Roanoke Rapids mills at a lower salary because of his sense of family responsibility, and worked there a total of twenty years, but was declared ineligible for a pension because he didn't work ten *consecutive* years for J. P. Stevens. The company did present him with a box of towels.

Although mild and articulate, Bud describes his experience in bitter terms. "For a man who has been through [what] I have in Germany . . . and having seen those concentration camps, you have to train your mind to put that in the past, but when you see . . . this going on, you got to stop a little bit, that such things can get to be that bad." After years of hard work at low wages, after serving his nation and family with heroic loyalty, Bud Harrison found himself the victim of an occupational hoax. Company information about employees' breathing tests was never distributed and adequately explained, and when outside medical testimony definitively supported his claim, he was met with delay, conflict, attacks on his credibility, and on that very loyalty that pushed him to work when he was severely ill. "Not only have these people suffered in the mills, but once they became disabled and go through a period of sickness . . . before they are declared disabled by a doctor, they have had long sick periods. I was going to work and she [Louise] told me not to go."

Bud Harrison suffered another kind of penalty because textile workers are paid on a piece-work scale, that is, by the volume they produce. "You suffer twice because you worked less and earned less and when declared disabled, social security payments are less than they would have been." Bud now suffers from byssinosis, but is compensated for it. Because of Louise's early retirement, and his disability settlement, they both live on a social security payments. Bud's settlement was $16,000 in one lump sum. After paying legal fees and medical bills, his "compensation" for the loss of his lungs and a shortened, more painful life span amounted to less than one year's wages.

The hazardous conditions of mill work are enforced by an authoritarian management philosophy, even today. Workers fear for their jobs and are hesitant to speak publicly about plant conditions, but in private they offer detailed testimony of the intense dust and noise that continue to fill the mills. They cite numerous episodes of blatant intimidation by management against workers who speak out against the dangerous conditions. This authoritarian style of management has always been present in the mills, although it was less oppressive during the earlier years of the company when its policies were more paternalistic.

Mrs. Varnell Coates has experienced both types, and she described incidents characteristic of present-day management. In 1932, she began working in Roanoke Number One when she was twelve. Forty-five years later, she was declared a compensable byssinosis victim, but in the intervening years, her attempts to change work-place conditions were met with unequivocal resistance by her supervisors. In 1936, she was fired from her job for professing union sympathies. Consequently, she was blacklisted. After repeated attempts to regain employment, she was turned down while others with less experience were hired. Mrs. Coates went to the general manager of the then Simmons plant (now J. P. Stevens). She asked why she wasn't allowed to work. He said, "What do you think of the union now, I stopped and thought for a minute . . . and I said if you had a union I wouldn't ask for a job . . . and the next day, I got called to go to work. But when the union came again and when the union passed, I voted for it. [J. P. Stevens] didn't know what I was thinking. I didn't let my right hand know what my left was doing." In the case of Mrs. Coates, the conjunction of company power and governmental cooperation prevented her from joining her fellow workers to demand a healthier work place. The union was voted in in 1975. Her breathing capacity is well below normal for her age—her damaged lungs are the price of her employment.

Greenville, South Carolina

Greenville is the textile center of the Carolinas. It is a city that has declared itself the "anti-union" capital of the South. Although it is small in population (62,000 in the city and approximately 300,000 in the county), it is significant as a center of anti-union and conservative politics. It is the home of J. P. Stevens, Michelin Tire, Bob Jones University, Nixon's Supreme Court nominee Clement Haynsworth, and Roger Milliken, head of Deering-Milliken, the largest privately owned textile firm. It wasn't until 1960 that a state law prohibiting blacks from working in the industry was declared unconstitutional. In 1977, the local business and political elite successfully opposed the introduction of a large Phillip Morris plant in Greenville because of the tobacco company's contract with the Tobacco workers' Union.

Greenville is part of the South Carolina political and economic heritage: in 1980, South Carolina ranked 43rd among states in percentage of families with incomes under $3,000; 42nd in number of hospital beds per one thousand persons; 48th in average student-teacher ratio; 49th in the percentage of the work force unionized; 47th in the average industrial wage; 47th in per capita welfare assistance; and 46th in per capita personal income.[5]

These harsh statistics do not reveal the human suffering caused by South Carolina's textile politics. The impact of these cold statistics on the ordinary people of South Carolina can be better understood by reviewing the work history of Paul Cline, a 58-year-old disabled textile worker suffering from byssinosis. He is a proud, conservative man who feels victimized by a system of political and economic power that routinely considered the welfare of textile workers and other citizens an afterthought in their obsession with preserving the paternalistic cultural and economic status quo that defined life in the South since the Civil War.

The Cline family employment in the textile industry dates to Paul's grandfather, a small sharecropper, who was recruited by a labor agent of a mill. "Back then they painted a pretty picture. People on a farm only got paid once a year but in textiles you got paid every week, and that kind of looked good to people on a farm who didn't make much. They tried it." Eight Clines joined as a group, including Paul's grandfather, his uncles, and his father. The children were between seven to ten years old at the time. "My daddy started off sweepin' and cleanin' mills. He was eight years old. They put the paycheck into one, the head of the house. I believe my dad made ten cents a day. They would buy their groceries from the company store. We did like that and my dad and mom married and had five kids, each in a different mill."

Paul's father was an individualist who believed in preserving a degree of self-respect and autonomy on the job. He didn't conform to the deferential work culture demanded by textile foremen and paternalistic mill owners. Consequently his work history was characterized by conflicts and moves from one textile mill town to another. "They used to say we had an old rooster when it seen a wagon comin' it knowed it was time to move, it just laid down and crossed its legs because my daddy was goin' to move again. He was high tempered. He wouldn't take no stuff off of them."

Paul began his life in the mills like his father, but the majority of his work history is characterized by diligence, productivity, and obedience. In 1975, his world changed and his understanding of his own history was altered dramatically. "It is honest work and people [were] dedicated to their companies. You could meet up with people just like I did and a whole lot more who worked just practically all their lives and got cotton dust and [were] treated dirty. It is just unreasonable a corporation that big [J. P. Stevens] could treat the people that helped make their money that way."

Paul began working in the mills in the 1930s and he was drafted into military service in 1943. He returned to the mill and worked with cotton as well as fiberglass and asbestos in making still mill uniforms for furnace work. "I didn't know I had it in my lungs until I went to the hospital for a bladder operation in 1975. The doctor called me into his office and wanted to know if I worked in a fiber glass plant and this stunned me because he didn't know my background. 'Sure,' I said, 'how did you know that.' He said he wanted to ask another question. 'Did you work on asbestos?' I was still stunned. I said I sure did. He said, 'We just took some x-rays and its still in your lungs.' I said that has been 15 years ago. But I got better and I still went back to the mill." Shortly after, the company doctor who diagnosed the fiber glass and asbestos in Paul Cline's lungs was released by the textile firm.

But Mr. Cline's doctor insisted that Paul leave the mills and declared a leave of absence for him. "The company got real mad. I could not have got fired if I laid out. They fired a lot of people that way. I drew $75 a week in private insurance. After six months it ran out. I had nothing." Mr. Cline wasn't 62 and the local Social Security office declared him eligible for work even though four doctors wrote in support of his disability application. He appealed that decision to a regional office and won the hearing a year later. In the interim, he exhausted his personal savings.

A short time later Mrs. Cline was referred to the Brown Lung Association by its local branch. The BLA administered a breathing test to both of them. At the age of 56, Paul Cline only had 57 percent of his breathing capacity. His wife, a life-long textile worker, had 55 percent. They joined the Carolina Brown Lung Association (CBLA) and pursued a compensation award. Both disabled and old before their time, they encountered grueling medical tests and travel in order to satisfy the Stevens' insurance representative, Liberty Mutual. They accepted an "out of court" settlement, a lump sum disability payment without future coverage for medical costs. "I didn't know how long I was going to last so I took the money instead of fighting a long compensation case." After 38 years in the mills, he received $22 a month pension from Stevens. Yet Paul Cline will tell you, "Textile people down here are proud people. They give it all. They don't want charity. They'd rather work. I want to work. I took pride in my work. I'm proud of being a textile worker . . . I don't want to see nobody lose their jobs. I just want to see the mills cleaned up because somewhere down the line these people are goin' to get sick and I don't want them to get what we got. I want my lungs back." Conditions in the textile industry are still unhealthy. "I got some grandchildren starting out working in the same place I started out and they haven't cleaned it up one bit."

Anderson, South Carolina

The brown lung legacy of the Carolinas is composed of numerous cases of social injustice and industrial negligence like those of Paul Cline and Bud Harrison, and all the others in Roanoke Rapids. Many cases go unrecorded because brown lung victims are diagnosed as emphysema patients and so never know the occupational cause of their disease. They die prematurely and their deaths, erroneously, are not linked to cotton dust and textile industry negligence. But even a random survey of textile centers and mill towns in the Carolinas will yield many tragic histories of hard work, authoritarian management, low wages, and mistreatment by the compensation system.

On November 7, 1979, I visited the local CBLA office in Anderson, South Carolina and met Fred Dowkins, sixty-four years old, who was general overseer (foreman) in the cloth room and a textile worker for over fifty years. He was joined by Frank Lackey, a fifty-six-year-old disabled textile worker, employed since 1946, and Neal Powell, sixty years old and a textile veteran of thirty-five years, twenty-eight with J. P. Stevens. During our three-hour talk, they each coughed and hacked their way through the interview in the storefront office.

Fred Dowkins isn't supposed to be injured by faulty management. He was management. As an overseer, he was a shop-floor supervisor participating directly in the production process. Two years before his retirement he realized that he had a serious breathing problem. His acceptance of his managerial responsibilities had led him to implicitly trust company policy regarding work-place health. From fourteen years of age, Mr. Dowkins labored in the spooling room, the roller shop, the carding room, and the weave room. He worked for fifteen years in the finishing shop before his last sixteen years as an overseer in the cloth room. How could his superiors be lax regarding *his* health since he was part of *their* control of the plant? It wasn't until the distinguished Yale expert on byssinosis, Dr. Arend Bouhuys, diagnosed his condition as brown lung that Fred Dowkins began to understand the reality of his years of loyal company service. He now has begun a compensation case for byssinosis. Unless state and federal laws are changed to permit a "presumptive diagnosis," Mr. Dowkins faces a lengthy battle, pitting his life expectancy against the corporate, insurance, and governmental interests in a drawn-out hearing process.

Neal Powell faced a similar future. Although a hospital diagnosis warned him that he has byssinosis in a mild stage, the local social security office has rejected his claim for social security compensation (a separate entitlement from workmen's compensation). In his thirty-five years in the mills, Mr. Powell experienced coughing fits but they were always diagnosed by his family physician as bronchitis. On occasion, J. P. Stevens conducted breathing tests for its employees, but the company did not release the results. Mr. Powell was never given critical information about his coughing problem by the company even though he was tested by them.

It wasn't until a nurse at Stevens subtly suggested to him that he see a doctor concerning his "bronchitis" and its link to the mill that Mr. Powell was led to suspect an occupational connection to what he always believed was a unique personal health problem. In 1978, a doctor diagnosed his condition as byssinosis and strongly advised him to leave the mill. He was fifty-nine years old. Mr. Powell would lose $700 in vacation pay if he retired immediately. He continued to work from January until July and then he retired. "I coughed . . . I get guys that worked by me and they kept telling me, 'Mr. Powell there is something wrong with you, you're coughing too much.' I just take a spell and cough, go over in a corner and cough and cough. And I didn't smoke neither. I didn't smoke for over 23 years."

When Neal Powell discussed the diagnosis with J. P. Stevens management, he was met with skepticism and aloofness. "My bossman, I mentioned it to him and he said to me, 'You don't have no brown lung. There is no such thing. You may have a lung problem.'" The refusal of the textile companies to recognize brown lung directly relates to their refusal to seriously redress the problem in the workplace both by fighting all byssinosis compensation claims, and by fiercely resisting the new OSHA regulation for cotton dust at every available administrative and legal level.

Sitting patiently while Fred Dowkins and Neal Powell discussed their disabilities, Frank Lackey seemed composed and not hesitant to discuss his personal experiences with the mills and the compensation system. It wasn't until I asked several questions that I realized that Frank Lackey was unable to hear me or the others. For most of his thirty-two years in the mills, he worked in the noisiest area in textile plants, the weave room.

He was diagnosed as a byssinosis victim in 1978, and tried, unsuccessfully, to continue on his job. He then attempted to work in a variety of other shops, but his failing lungs and severe hearing loss presented insurmountable obstacles. He had lost 71 percent of his hearing and 69 percent of his breathing capacity. For thirty years of underpaid factory work, he has a double disability at age fifty-six, and faces long and tense hearings if he hopes to win compensation from the South Carolina Industrial Commission.

Because of Frank's pride and strong work ethic, he tried the mills again even though he was advised by his physician to cease all work. He took a job in the Anderson mill on the third shift (12–8 A.M.). "It was time to go home, it was pitiful. The shape I was in when I came out that morning because everybody else left and I thought I was going to die. I said to myself that if I ever made it home I don't believe I'd ever make another night. I laid down on the couch all that day and night. It took a week to get over it. Later a specialist diagnosed it as brown lung, but the general hospital said there was nothing wrong and knocked me out of my social security and everything. My family doctor and a specialist both said I could never go back, and I hadn't smoked since 1957."

The politics of the compensation apparatus have made it extremely difficult and debilitating for the Frank Lackeys of the Carolinas to ever receive even an *inadequate* monetary compensation for brown lung. With several physicians concurring, one a lung specialist, Frank Lackey was told to return to mill work although he had suffered 70 percent losses in hearing and breathing capacity. Furthermore, he was not compensated for either his hearing loss or brown lung from the social security administration. He was asked to choose between a modest income or his health. His only source of funds was his veterans benefits, which he earned from his military service. His family suffered with him.

Conclusion

The textile legacy of brown lung disease may appear to be an aberration of industrial relations in the United States, but it is far from that. Deaths caused by occupational health and safety hazards number over 100,000 annually, and even with a more efficient and responsive OSHA, this number may increase as the number of lethal chemicals used in the work place increases beyond the limits of regulatory control.[6] The tragic histories of illness and death in the mining of uranium, talc, zinc, copper, and coal, join those of the textile industry. The many workplaces affected by the production, use, and general exposure of workers to asbestos remains significant in number. The exposure of hundreds of thousands of workers to carcinogenic chemicals in the auto, steel, aluminum, smelting, and chemical industries means that the compensation system probably has and will not recognize hundreds and thousands of deaths as occupationally related, because of the long latency period of so many occupational diseases. Any serious attempt to redress the health crisis in the workplace requires a preventive approach to the problem. It is this need for prevention that led to the creation of OSHA. But now, OSHA finds itself confronted with a pro-business assault on its very existence. Anti-regulation proponents direct their fire at OSHA's preventive policies so that proposed reforms of the OSHA act will reverse the preventive orientation of the agency and restore the traditional compensatory approach to the problem of work-place health and safety. No other conclusion can be drawn but that the compensation system will result in unnecessary death and illness, compromised political and bureaucratic administration, and restoration of the previous corporate policy of "work now and grieve later." As the biographies of Bud Harrison, Paul Cline, Mrs. Coates, and other textile workers recorded in this essay testify, a change in OSHA practices means making the worker fit the workplace. This is not technology serving the worker, but rather labor serving profit.

The objectionable aspect of OSHA for business management has little to do with bureaucratic red tape and the "unproductive" investment of regulatory compulsion. It is not environmental regulation that is causing lower levels of productivity in basic American industry, but the economics of old plants and poor engineering coupled with the needs of multinational companies to have diversified portfolios and to consolidate capital. The decisions of American steel companies to invest in chemicals and oil rather than in new plants accounts, in large part, for declining productivity in the steel industry. Declining productivity and profits in the American automobile industry seem to be more a function of management decisions and engineering timidity than a result of over-spending on pollution controls required by OSHA or the EPA. In fact, the Japanese automobile industry, a very successful competitor against the American producer, spends a greater amount on environmental regulation than its American counterpart.

The anti-regulation politics of the business community is an attempt to maximize its managerial discretion while continuing to preserve authoritarian control over its workforce. The attempt to limit or abolish OSHA is not so much a struggle over regulating investment as it is resistance to the sharing of responsibilities with workers, regardless of the limited extent of existing rights granted under OSHA. This is particularly evident in unionized industries like auto, steel, and chemicals. Here unions have succeeded, to some degree, in solidifying and extending worker rights to comply with OSHA regulations, for instance, in the use of full-time safety and health representatives on the shop floor. In the shadow of industrial and manufacturing decline in the U.S., even these advances remain problematic. The fear of job loss erodes all attempts to procure job rights. For the unorganized and less organized industries like textiles, the attack on OSHA limits worker initiatives in general. But in plants without unions, even the appearance of OSHA inspectors can lead directly to organizing around issues of occupational health and economic justice.

Even without the specter of anti-regulation activity, OSHA has a limited impact on the work place for several reasons. First, it always will be inferior in size and expertise to the number of companies that can oppose it. Second, the history of collective bargaining in the United States demonstrates the adversarial relationship between management and labor. Questions that compromise "management's right to manage" usually are avoided in favor of injury-compensation and work-rules issues. Although remarkable changes have occurred in some industries and unions, occupational health issues tend to have a lower priority than major questions of employment and injury compensation. Consequently, the enforcement of OSHA regulations and initiatives for new regulations are reduced. This is the reality of workplace politics in unionized industries, with several exceptions such as the Oil Chemical and Atomic Workers (OCAW), the United Auto Workers (UAW), and, to a growing degree, the United Steel Workers of America (USWA). Even in these unions, the record of enforcement varies by union locals and specific contract provisions.

The third restraint on OSHA's effectiveness is the very nature of the political economy. OSHA and its constituents represent only one aspect of the complex of regulatory and executive branch politics. The economic impact of OSHA is challenged by competing agencies and interests in and around the White House. Any specific proposed regulation will encounter some resistance by the Council of Economic Advisors, the Office of Management and Budget, and ad hoc groups appointed by the White House. In short, the dominant political and economic interests in the United States will structurally limit efforts to extend environmental regulations. Increased inflation, costs to specific industries, and higher unemployment will be cited as reasons for opposition.

The consequence of OSHA's limitations and the legacy of the injury-compensation system, in the face of an increasing number of expanding workplace hazards and greater knowledge about them, results in a significant increase in occupational illness and death. The growing health crisis of the workplace will continue unless there is a dramatic alteration in the approach to work-place regulation in the United States. Without the continued extension of worker rights and participation in occupation health and safety regulation, the probability of a more severe crisis looms. The limts on OSHA and the present political mood of anti-regulation restricts the future of the agency. All future public policy regarding health and safety will be ineffective without a viable OSHA.

Whether or not increased worker participation will be the future course of occupational safety and health policy in the United States is dependent on several factors. First, the conceptualization of the work process significantly conditions the expectations and demands that are made on it. The ideology of work in the public consciousness affects the future of health and safety. Second, the political economy of regulation will significantly shape the choices available on the shop floor. The politics of OSHA, the posture and influence of organized labor, the strength and character of a broader safety and health movement (one including health professionals, activists, and public interest organizations), and the responsiveness of workers themselves dictates workplace politics. The counterpart to these initiatives includes managerial decisions as well as international and domestic economic factors affecting capital formation, investment, and productivity levels. Public policy formation is not just an activity between the regulatory agency and the respective industry, but rather it requires a complex interplay of economic, political, and cultural interests that presume a "politics from below" as well as one from above. Whether disabled workers will be an increasing phenomenon on the American industrial landscape, is the consequence of these choices.

NOTES

1. Deposition of Joseph M. Bosworth, M.D. in *Wilkins* vs. *Lanier*. Civil Action No. CV–79–294 in the Circuit Court of Lee County, Alabama, June 9, 1983, pp. 88–90.

2. "Brown Lung: Case of Deadly Neglect," *Charlotte Observer*, February 3, 1980. An excellent accounting of the incidence of brown lung disease in the Carolina textile industry is available in a telling eight-part series written for the *Charlotte Observer*, February 3–10, 1980.

3. "Stevens Mill Workers Protest Their Lack of a Contract," *The New York Times*, August 8, 1979, p. A–13.

4. Presumptive diagnosis means workers seeking eligibility for workmen's compensation will be "presumed" to be disabled by virtue of their experience in a recognized hazardous occupation.

5. For an interesting and detailed historical and political overview of Greenville, South Carolina, see Cliff Sloan and Bob Hall, "It's Good to Be Home in Greenville," *Southern Exposure*, vol. 7, no. 1 (Spring 1979).

6. *The President's Report on Occupational Safety and Health* (Washington, D.C.: U.S. Government Printing Office, 1972), p. 111.

7 / *Manslaughter in a Coal Mine*

HARRY M. CAUDILL

DIGGING COAL is hard and ruinous work. Even strip-mining, which now accounts for half the nation's output, takes its inexorable human toll. But it is underground that coal mining reaches its deadly worst. In the long tunnels leading to the working areas, at the dust-choked "face" where machines rend the hard bituminous rock from the vein, and along the tracks and conveyor belts by which the fuel is carried to the outside, accidents occur with numbing frequency. The perils are legion. In the cramped confines of the mines the huge machines mangle bodies with the efficiency of sausage grinders. Roofs crash down despite wooden props and steel bolts. Poorly managed blasting snuffs out lives. Coal and rock dust suspended in the air that must be breathed cause slow strangulation from pneumoconiosis and silicosis. Most dramatic of all, methane gas can seep from the coal veins and blow up with a violence approaching that of gunpowder.

For most of the nation's history its coal mines operated in remote areas, received little attention from law makers and the public, and derived such safety standards as existed from feeble state mining bureaus and the well-sheltered consciences of mine owners. The former were always short of funds and routinely staffed by persons "friendly to the industry"; the latter could rarely abide safety procedures because they cost money and cut into profits. Consequently, miners died in small numbers, and large, crippled ex-miners limped along the streets of coal towns; by 1968 nearly 250,000 men were gasping, half-dead victims of pneumoconiosis, and half as many more had already been sent to inconspicuous graves by the same deadly ailment. A hundred thousand had died in mining accidents since the industry began.

Then on November 20, 1968 Consolidation Coal Company's mine at Fairmont, W. Va., blew up, killing seventy-eight men. There had been deadlier mine catastrophes in U.S. history—362 miners died at Monongah, W. Va., in 1907—but this was spectacular and television played it to the hilt, startling millions of viewers with the immense eruptions of black smoke that roared from the pit-head and drifted over the somber hills. The Governor rushed to the scene, to be photographed looking solemn and sympathetic, and used the opportunity to point out that mining is inherently dangerous, but that Consolidation had an unusually fine safety record. W. A. Boyle, then president of the United Mine Workers, mouthed similar nonsense. "Consol" was part and parcel of the U.S. coal industry, its largest producer and general pace setter, and it shared fully in the industry's disgraceful casualty figures.

Sen. Harrison Williams of New Jersey took the lead in drafting and enacting legislation designed to prevent similar calamities. The Appalachian mining states were represented by influential legislators who might have been expected to initiate this legislation. But coal companies are so powerful in West Virginia, Kentucky, Virginia, Tennessee, Pennsylvania and Alabama, and coal miners and their families are so politically inert, that the elected representatives from the region deemed it the better part of valor to leave the work to other hands. In any event, the time for a new law had come. The Federal Coal Mine Health and Safety Act of 1969 entered the U.S. Code, and two extremely reluctant Presidents—first Nixon, then Ford—took up the task of implementing it. The Mine Enforcement and Safety Administration (MESA) was created and charged to enforce the new safety code.

Thus for the first time the federal government undertook to rein in and civilize the vast, fragmented, widely dispersed and still ideologically laissez-faire coal industry. Largely centered in Appalachia, where individualism and distrust of government are rampant, the industry's managers fully reflect these attitudes—and so do their employees. The chaotic conditions within coal can be measured by a comparison of fatality ratios per million manshifts worked underground in the ten years following World War II. Bear in mind that European mines were ravaged by that war, while U.S. mines were ravaged only by mismanagement and lack of foresight.

In Great Britain the death rate ranged from 0.44 in 1947 to 0.24 in 1954. In Belgium it declined from 0.66 in 1947 to 0.32 in 1955. In France the rate dropped from 0.48 in 1948 to 0.34 in 1955. In West Germany the figures went from a high of 0.77 in 1948 to 0.61 in 1955. In Holland, which almost certainly operates the world's safest pits, the fatality rate fell from a high of 0.53 to 0.15. In the United States during the same interval the high was 1.22 in 1947 and the low was 0.84 in 1952.

These data reflect a general unconcern with safety and lives that persisted with only minimal change through the Great Crusade, the New Frontier and the Great Society. That unconcern permitted the methane buildup along the miles of dusty, coal-black tunnels at Fairmont and culminated in the colossal explosion that roared with such deadly force under the West Virginia hills.

Gordon Bonnyman is 57, a slender man with restraint stamped in every line of his spare frame. He is one of the vanishing breed of American businessmen who have managed to hold onto inherited wealth and expand it for the next generation. The Bonnymans have left their everlasting mark on the torn and battered Appalachian landscape. The map reflects the names of their old operations at Bonnyman, Ky., and Bonny Blue, Va. Their new operations are conducted by Blue Diamond Coal Co. in the eastern Kentucky hills.

Blue Diamond is controlled and largely owned by Bonnyman and his family, and they do not give out information concerning stockholders and dividends. But in 1976 *Forbes* magazine reported that in 1975 Blue Diamond had increased its liquid assets by $55.4 million, that it had in fact enriched its treasury by $150,000 per day throughout a year that most Americans recall as the most depressed in three decades. Nor is there any reason to suppose that the cornucopia ceased to flow as spring drew near in 1976.

Scotia Coal Co., a wholly owned subsidiary of Blue Diamond, generated more than a third of the profits *Forbes* had found so remarkable. Operating in thick, hard veins of heat-rich metallurgical coal in Letcher County, Kentucky, its strip mines and endless outpourings of wastes have done much to ruin a once beautiful tributary of the Cumberland River. But this immensely profitable mine was not without serious problems. The stripping operation attacked only the forest-heavy outcrops of the vein: tunnels followed the coal thousands of yards into the immense ridge.

In March 1976, Scotia's operations were about typical of at least half the nation's soft coal producers. No one connected in any way with the management of the company displayed any visible concern for land, air or water. They regarded environmentalists as nuts. To them the United Mine Workers of America with its royalty-supported Health and Welfare Fund was anathema, and the federal program to compensate disabled black-lung victims was a "give-away." The poor people huddled in the hollows were disdained. Watching University of Kentucky basketball games on television was their most coveted form of entertainment, and the overriding goal of right thinking people was to dig coal and make money. The miners on their payrolls shared most of these views, seeing nothing wrong with the arrangements per se, but inclining to the notion that they should collect larger chunks of the profit pie. Their share was already quite good. To keep them from being lured into the UMW, Scotia paid wages substantially higher than those received at unionized pits. Wages began at $52 per light-hour shift for the lowest categories and went to $64 for skilled machine operators. There was plenty of overtime, which drew 50 percent more. Generally the men worked six days a week, and sometimes on Sunday. There was a cash bonus of 10 percent for those who missed no workdays in a month. Thus wages ran from $12,000 to $16,000 and a few miners with a lust for work and no regard for Sundays or holidays boasted of $30,000 in 1975. Fringe benefits were meager, but they were of little interest to Scotia's 400 miners, most of whom were young and expected that pension funds—including Social Security—would "go broke" long before they reached retirement age.

For all this munificence Scotia demanded one thing: coal. It must clatter through the tipple and fill the railroad cars all day and all night, shift after shift, irrespective of injuries, pneumoconiosis, bad weather or state and federal safety laws.

On March 9, 1976, the third shift began as usual. The solemn enactments of Congress and the state legislature, and the regulations adopted pursuant thereto, provide the manner in which a new shift of workmen shall take place and the precautions that must be observed for their survival. Such laws and regulations are sound enough, but what actually happened on that ill-fated shift demonstrates the leaden inability of state and federal bureaucracies to carry public mandates into effect.

Charlie Fields a short, plump, red-faced man whose physical appearance betrays many years in the air-short, dust-abundant mines. His breath comes in the labored gasps of incipient emphysema and black lung. Ambitious beyond most miners, he improved his lot by studying for the "mining papers" of a foreman. Because of a meager education this had come hard for him, especially the meaning of engineering terms used in the state's written examination. But his perseverance and ambition were rewarded and Charlie was eventually employed by Scotia to "fire-boss" the third shift. It is clear that he took his duties lightly, but there is scant reason to suppose he was appreciably less conscientious than most of his fellows similarly engaged in the industry. Perhaps he simply failed to appreciate the seriousness of the task with which he, as a licensed foreman, was charged by law.

It is the duty of a fire boss or "pre-shift safety examiner" to inspect all working places and all haulways leading into them within a three-hour span before a work shift begins. He must see that air circulation meets the required norms and that roof conditions are safe. He is expected to detect fire hazards, including such obvious risks as spark-emitting machinery, improperly stored combustibles of all kinds, accumulations of coal dust, and, most importantly and obviously, the presence of methane. The caged canary has long since disappeared and a methanometer now gives accurate readings of the percentage of the gas in the air. Methane becomes explosive at 5 percent and ceases to be explosive at 15 percent. Prudent supervisors are likely to empty a section when 0.75 percent methane is detected, the men being kept out until new airflows remove the gas.

At the official hearings held at the courthouse in the county seat two months later, it was made clear that Charlie Fields did not inspect that portion of the mine known as No. 2-Southeast Main, though he had entered in the log or journal that he had checked the area and that no gas was detected. When questioned by Robert Barrett, director of MESA on April 27, 1976, he admitted that the entry could have been erroneous. Someone had told him that the air was good and he had accepted that assurance as adequate and entered a notation that the ventilation was 14,300 cubic feet per minute at the last "open cross-cut" in the "straight" of 2-Southeast Main. That is an immense volume of fresh air, surely enough to dilute to harmlessness any methane it encounters.

Fields conceded that he rarely made any inspections, relying instead on a subordinate, Arvil Cornett, to do so. On the basis of Cornett's reports to him he then made the log entries that constituted the mine's official record. He had been to the straight of 2-Southeast Main only twice in six weeks, though he knew of a "gas feeder" in that inactive dead-end tunnel that emitted such volumes that concentrations had risen to at least 5 percent at one time. He did not recall reporting that discovery. He had been instructed by higher level management to sign the log routinely on the basis of Cornett's reports.

As for Cornett, he told the hearing officers that he too had failed to inspect the long section at the end of the heading because he did not expect anyone to enter it. According to some miners who knew the area, brattices—barriers to shunt air from the fans to working places—had routed the oxygen to this new section, leaving 600 yards at the end of 2-Southeast Main temporarily abandoned and sealed off behind the brattice curtains. Even without these fixtures, air, following the line of least resistance, would enter the new section rather than push into the dead-end tunnel straight ahead. Thus the air in the idle length of tunnel was undisturbed as the days passed.

Then, on March 9, a crew from the third shift was directed to haul a load of tract rails into the section, preparatory to bringing in a new "continuous miner." The inspection log showed the section to be free of gas and adequately ventilated, so two workmen blithely drove two electric locomotives, with their carloads of steel rails, into an arena no methanometer had entered for at least a day and probably a month. Cornett noted that at the entry to the new branch tunnel he had found the air flow to be 10,120 cubic feet of air per minute, 30 percent less than was stated in the log. He had "heard rumors" of a methane feeder, but had not tried to track them down.

Just before the locomotive appeared in the area, problems had developed in the new working area, identified by the engineers on their maps as "2-left off 2-Southeast Main." The air was "bad" and there was "not enough" of it, according to miners, who said that Virgil Coots, the 23-year-old-foreman, telephoned this information to James Bentley, ventilation foreman. Bentley, who had countersigned Charlie Field's log, denied that any such call was received, and testified that someone unknown to him and without authority to do so had opened an air regulator 4 feet. When this happened, Coots called to say "he had lost it [the air]."

Two minutes later fifteen men died as an immense, booming ball of fire streaked out of the far limits of 2-Southeast Main, swept 1,800 feet to the entrance of 2-left off 2-Southeast Main, and flashed into it with a searing roar. The locomotives with the track layers had ventured into the long-deserted section and their arrival had set off gas accumulations that no one had bothered to suspect.

The Scotia mine had been inspected hundreds of times before March 9, 1976, and 652 violations of safety laws and regulations had been cited. Of these at least sixty infractions dealt with serious ventilation problems, including insufficient air circulating at the working face, line brattices out of position, inoperative methanometers, failure to follow the ventilation plan, and findings of imminent danger of explosions, due to methane concentrations of 1.2 percent. Penalties amounting to $164,352 had been imposed by assessment officers, but the company had actually paid only $78,877.

Neither the mine superintendent, the general foreman nor the vice president in immediate charge of the operation regularly checked on the work of the fire bosses or made routine inspections on their own initiative. As one of them put it, "Everybody knew what he was supposed to do and we just left it up to him to do it."

As for Gordon Bonnyman, who lives 150 miles away in Knoxville, he said that he knew nothing of any safety violations. At the courthouse hearings he described Blue Diamond as "a small, informally structured operation" that ran three coal mines in Kentucky and clay and mica mines in North Carolina. His time was spent at the Knoxville headquarters and from his demeanor and testimony one could surely conclude that the goings-on in the tunnels under Big Black Mountain were as remote to him as the harvesting procedures in Bulgaria.

The haphazard management practices at Scotia were matched by the equally haphazard and erratic conditions in the regional and Washinton offices of MESA. As soon as he heard the news of the explosion, Herschel Potter, chief of the Division of Safety for MESA in the region, proclaimed that "Scotia stands tall in the industry" in matters of mine safety; he then rushed to the scene. There he met Robert Barrett, director of MESA, who had flown down from Washington with a covey of unimpressive looking "experts." After solemn conferences with company "management teams" and representatives of the anemic Scotia Employees' Association, a recovery team recruited from other mining companies brought out the dead bodies. It had not yet been discovered where the explosion originated or what had set it off, but coal production must go on "in these energy-short times" so, in the same shambling fashion, a crew was organized to go in and restore air circulation and rebolt the blast-weakened roof. This crew of men was accompanied by three MESA inspectors who were to see that the work was properly performed under the immediate supervision of foreman Don Polly. This time the "fire-bossing" was done by a MESA inspector and another company foreman. The former had no anamometer or carbon monoxide monitor. Incredibly, one of the workmen, P.D. Holbrook, was a machinist with absolutely no underground mining experience! The preposterous decision to include him in the crew was concurred in by MESA, the company, and the miners' "association." Toward the end of their shift a laconic notation was entered in MESA's log: "All O.K."

By then Barrett had flown back to Washington where, a few hours later, on March 11, he was confronted with the doleful news that another explosion had ripped out of that same deadly tunnel. This time eleven were killed, including all three of the MESA men.

Barrett and his experts reassembled at the gloom-and-doom shrouded mine where the lethargy at all levels had begun somewhat to dissolve.

A session of buck-passing and recriminations now ensued, as the company and the miners' association blamed MESA for the twin calamities, while the undaunted bureaucrats placed the entire responsibility squarely on the company.

At this point MESA began to formulate a theory to explain the blasts. It seems that one of the battery-powered locomotives, used to transport the steel rails into 2-Southeast Main, was equipped with pneumatic brakes instead of the usual manual type. A compressor automatically pumped up the pressure of these brakes at half-hour intervals, and each time this occurred it set off what was variously described as an electric "arc," "spark" or "flash." It was postulated that, when this machine was driven into the temporarily abandoned 2-Southeast Main section, the compressor ignited the accumulated methane. This kind of brake was a rarity necessitated by the uneven floor of the mine, so, quite naturally, MESA did not suspect its existence. The locomotive was still in the section, but the company did not inform MESA about the arc-producing mechanism, which would continue to function at half-hour intervals for weeks, until the battery was exhausted. Thus, the theory ran, MESA, misled by the company's silence, allowed the roof bolters and its own supervisors to enter a gassy pit in which a "possible ignition source" functioned every half hour. For a time this afforded MESA a tenuous escape hatch and it was clung to with the fervor of a drowning man holding to a life float.

Eventually the mine was sealed at all its openings to allow the air to "stabilize" and the battery to expire. It was reopened in July and miners working in oxygen respirators spent two months restoring brattices, pumping out immense pools of water, restoring electrical and telephone lines and shoring up the top. The bodies were reached and brought out in late November.

The Scotia explosions graphically illustrate all that is wrong with the nation's coal mines. The gritty work of running the pits has been delegated to low-echelon foremen and superintendents of mediocre competence, and frequently, slight education. Top management avoids the tipples and tunnels and knows little about the guts of the operation. Management at the mine level delegates responsibility ever downward to foremen and sub-foremen, of whom there are seldom enough. For example, if Charlie Fields had lawfully "fire-bossed" the fatal third shift, he would have traveled more than 5 miles and stopped for inspections at dozens of working places, an obvious impossibility. The miners are hooked on high wages and resent any action that might cost them a shift. They are untrained for their dangerous work and few, even among the experienced, have any real understanding of the dangers they must encounter. In their ignorance on the one hand and greed on the other, they virtually court disaster. As for MESA, it is staffed with "experts" who know little more than the miners (from whose ranks they are recruited) and, like Herschel Potter, instinctively react in defense of the industry they theoretically police. And when a company increases its liquid assets by $55.4 million in a single year how can its anti-social propensities be checked by penalties totaling $78,877 or, for that matter, $164,352?

The corporation that drew such prompt encomiums from Potter had wholly omitted to educate its miners in safety procedures. Some of the men said they had never been shown how to put on a "self-rescue" respirator, designed to make survival possible in pits from which fire or explosion has removed the oxygen. They had been taught nothing about the geology of the mountain in which they worked and had no understanding of the nature of methane or the huge "kettle bottom" rocks that can drop with silent deadliness out of the roof. Methane escapes in increasing quantities as barometric pressures fall, but the mine did not even own a barometer. The mine had no rescue teams, trained to enter disaster areas and bring out survivors. It had never staged escape drills. The company did not keep an ambulance to carry injured miners to hospitals, the nearest of which was 15 miles away over a narrow and extremely winding road. When the men asked that one be bought, the company said it would put up half the cost, and the miners could pay the balance. Under these circumstances, hundreds of men were sent as far as 2.5 miles into a ridge that towered above their heads for thousands of feet, the twisted strata propped up on coal pillars and wooden beams, and strung together with tenuous steel bolts or pins. Such a ramshackle situation made catastrophe almost inevitable.

To a considerable extent the hearings into the March 1976 blasts were taken up with testimony of miners concerning the loose day-to-day operation of the mine. There were accounts of MESA-ordered ventilation curtains being routinely taken down during the working shift so as not to impede the passage of "shuttle cars," then rehung to impress inspectors expected with the fresh work crews. A continuous litany told of advance warning that MESA inspectors were on their way, whereupon all hands flew to making the mine passable. In such instances, it was reported, electrical facilities were quickly insulated, defective methane detectors were replaced, conveyor belts were cleaned up, and ventilation systems were put in order. Though company spokesmen denied it, some of the miners insisted that ventilation regulators were reset to keep bountiful air flowing in areas undergoing inspection, the excellent circulation accompanying inspectors as they moved from section to section. Meanwhile, stale air was the lot of the men whose areas had already met the eye of the "Secretary's representatives." This insidious and deadly game of cat and mouse continued, according to their accounts, right up to the fatal shift.

As it turned out MESA could not shelter for long behind a plea of ignorance concerning those arc-emitting brakes. At the agency's hearings Ben Taylor, chief of the Whitesburg district office, admitted that a foreman had told him about the brake compressor and that he knew it generated an electrical arc. He discussed this with William Clemons, his superior, but Clemons dismissed the idea as unimportant. Neither mentioned the information to Robert Barrett, a newcomer to the position and a conscientious man, who sadly noted that he would never have authorized the roof-bolting crew to enter the mine if he had known of the compressor.

The two miners who survived the second explosion testified that the "MESA men," the foreman and some of the miners discussed the compressor and its periodic electrical arcing as they went into the mine, agreed that it could ignite still another blast, and then with the innocence of children playing with a cocked and loaded .45, proceeded straight on to a firey death a few hours later.

Neither Taylor nor Clemons has ever received any significant training in mine rescue work, and after the first explosion properly trained mine-rescue teams from nearby Bethlehem Steel and U.S. Steel operations had to be called in to bring out the fifteen bodies, this task being beyond the capacity of MESA and Kentucky's pitiable Department of Mines and Minerals.

This was too rich a field for Congressmen to avoid and in due time a hybrid group of Senators and Representatives came to Whitesburg for hearings. Chaired by Rep. Carl D. Perkins of the House Committee on Education and Labor, they spent six whole hours on a tragedy that had snuffed out twenty-six lives. They fulminated at the MESA personnel, solemnly and respectfully slapped the wrists of company spokesmen, and poured out immense flows of sympathy on the widows, orphans and other relatives of the dead who filled the chamber. As the hearings adjourned one of the widows said with a disconsolate shrug, "You can see from what went on here why people ain't got no faith in Washington nowadays."

No foreman was indicted or punished for neglect of duty. Thirteen months later no charges had been brought against Blue Diamond Coal, Scotia, Gordon Bonnyman, the MESA bureaucrats or anyone else. Twenty-six men died under circumstances that reek of carelessness, lack of skill, illegality, incompetence and official neglect, but no noteworthy changes have been induced by the tragedy. The same stockholders own the mine, which is operated under the same management and supervisory personnel. The surviving miners, their ranks fleshed out with eager new recruits, go on as before. The MESA personnel still come round on inspection tours and have issued more than 500 new citations for safety violations since those fatal days in March 1976. If sleepless nights have been endured it was because of profits lost during the months when the coal vein was sealed, not because outraged justice demanded retribution.

8 / Murder in the Workplace

NANCY FRANK

STEFAN GOLAB, a Polish immigrant, worked for Film Recovery Systems, Inc., a firm involved in recycling silver from used photographic plates. The recycling process used by Film Recovery involved soaking used X-ray plates in a cyanide solution. Golab and other workers in the Film Recovery plant "chipped the film, mixed the cyanide granules with water in the vats, stirred the chips in the potent mixture for three days with long rakes, scooped the spent—and cyanide soaked—film chips out of the vat with a giant vacuum cleaner, cleaned the tank in preparation for the next load, and scraped the silver from the terminal plates on which it had been recovered."

This recycling process is conducted safely by several firms across the country. Because of the dangers of cyanide, which is highly poisonous if swallowed, inhaled, or absorbed through the skin, workers must be protected with rubber gloves, boots, and aprons, respirators, and effective ventilation.

At the Film Recovery plant, however, these normal precautions were not taken. Workers were given only paper face masks and cloth gloves. Ventilation was so poor inside the plant that the air was thick with the odor of cyanide and a "yellowish haze" of cyanide fumes hung inside the plant. . . . Workers frequently became ill, going outside the plant to vomit, and then returning to their work over the fuming cyanide vats.

On February 10, 1985, Stefan Golab staggered from the cyanide tank he was working over, stumbled to the adjacent locker room, and collapsed. Some of his fellow workers dragged him outside and called an ambulance. When the ambulance arrived back at the hospital, Golab was dead. An autopsy was performed to determine the cause of death. When the medical examiner made the first incision, a strong almond-like smell came out of the body, indicating cyanide poisoning. Subsequent blood tests revealed that Golab had a blood cyanide level of 3.45 micrograms per milliliter, a lethal dose.

The autopsy findings led to an eight month investigation, resulting in the indictment of five Film Recovery executives on charges of murder and the indictment of Film Recovery Systems, Inc., and two related corporations on charges of manslaughter. Under Illinois law, "A person who kills an individual without lawful justification commits murder if, in performing the acts which cause the death . . . He knows that such acts create a strong probability of death or great bodily harm to that individual or another . . ." The indictment became the first recorded case of an employer being charged with murder for the work related death of an employee.

The investigation of Film Recovery Systems and subsequent court testimony revealed a grim scenario. A Cook County Hospital study of Golab's fellow workers, which was undertaken following his death, found that "at least two-thirds of Film Recovery's workers suffered ten times a month or more from each of four major symptoms of cyanide intoxication—dizziness, the taste of bitter almonds in the mouth, headaches and nausea and vomiting." . . . When workers complained to the foreman and plant manager about feeling ill, they were told to "go outside so you can have some fresh air."

Many workers were not aware that they were working with cyanide. According to a former bookkeeper for Film Recovery, illegal aliens were chosen to work in the plant. Because they could not read English, they could not read the warning labels on the drums of cyanide. Several employees observed skull-and-crossbones markings being painted or burned off the drums. Because company managers had never informed workers of the hazards of working with the chemical, workers who did see the skull-and-crossbones assumed that the chemical was dangerous only if it was swallowed. They did not know that it could be lethal if inhaled or absorbed through the skin.

At trial, the defense argued that conditions inside the plant were safe. Moreover, they argued, if it was unsafe, the defendants were not aware that it was unsafe. Finally, the defense argued that Golab died of causes unrelated to the plant conditions, challenging the medical examiner's findings and suggesting that perhaps Golab had eaten apple cores, and the cyanide in his blood came from the apple seeds. To corroborate the defendants' assertions that they did not believe that conditions in the plant were dangerous, defense counsel indicated that on several occasions the defendants had arranged to have family members work in the plant. The defense also noted that the plant had been given a "clean bill of health" by local and federal inspectors prior to Golab's death.

The failure of regulating agencies to discover the frightful conditions inside the Film Recovery plant is an unfortunate but interesting sidelight to this story. A federal OSHA inspector had visited the offices of Film Recovery, Inc., only two and one-half months before

Golab collapsed from cyanide poisoning. The inspector never conducted an inspection of the plant, however, because of Reagan administration guidelines which prohibit inspectors from conducting on-site inspections unless an examination of company safety records reveals a poor accident record.

Although Film Recovery employees were frequently sent home to rest when they became too dizzy and nauseated to work, the company's records indicated little lost time. Consequently, the inspector did not conduct an inspection of the plant. . . . In a subsequent inspection following Golab's death, OSHA issued two citations for lack of safety equipment and ultimately fined Film Recovery $2,425.

At the close of the trial, Judge Ronald J.D. Banks convicted three executives of murder and fourteen counts of reckless conduct, and convicted two corporations of involuntary manslaughter and fourteen counts of reckless conduct. In supporting his decision, Judge Banks found that . . .

. . . the conditions under which the workers in the plant performed their duties was [sic] totally unsafe. There was an insufficient amount of safety equipment on the premises. There were no safety instructions given to the workers. The workers were not adequately warned of the hazards and dangers of working with cyanide.

The judge also found that the three convicted defendants were "totally knowledgeable" of the hazards of cyanide. Judge Banks reiterated the evidence substantiating his finding that each of the three executives knew the dangers of cyanide and understood that their failure to provide proper protective equipment created a strong probability of death or great bodily harm. He continued:

Steven O'Neil [defendant and president of Film Recovery] testified . . . and I quote, "I was aware of all of the hazardous nature of cyanide." He knew hydrogen cyanide gas was present. He knew hydrogen cyanide gas, if inhaled, could be fatal.

Charles Kirschbaum [defendant and plant manager] saw workers vomiting. He was given a Material Safety Data Sheet. He read the label, and he knew what it said. He said that he did not wear the same equipment the workers did because he did not do the same work as the workers, even though he testified to the contrary.

Daniel Rodriguez [defendant and plant foreman] knew the workers got sick at the plant. He testified to that. He could read the label, and he read it manay times.

Each of the three defendants was sentenced to twenty-five years in prison and each corporation was fined $10,000. (One of the original five indicted executives successfully fought extradition from Utah and another had the charges against him dismissed halfway through the trial.)

The central issue presented by this case is whether, as a matter of policy, it is desirable to equate the behaviors of the Film Recovery executives with murder and to punish it as such. Commentators have referred to the charge of murder in this case as unprecedented, scary, and wild. Some commentators, such as Ralph Nader and Christopher Stone, hailed the verdict as an appropriate application of the criminal law. Nader applauded the verdict, saying, "There was a courageous prosecutor and a prudent judge who applied the law to the facts, irrespective of the fact that the defendants had three-piece suits." . . . Christopher Stone, an expert on corporate responsibility and corporate crime, commented, "I think this case will properly embolden prosecutors to bring corporate criminal cases, and other judges to stop looking the other way."

Others were more skeptical about the desirability of a murder conviction and expressed concern about how this verdict would change the traditional legal concept of murder. Richard Epstein, a University of Chicago Law School professor, noted, "One has had to show more than just knowledge of a risk of death, but also a hope or intent that the death would come to pass. Knowledge of risk has not been generally sufficient." He continued, commenting on the potential impact of the case, "There is the potential here, given the way most industrial accidents take place, that you'd have a credible shot of pursuing a murder case. It would present a very radical change, in nuance and practice, in the criminal law."

Perhaps the question should be put this way. Is there a difference between a murderer who exposed a person to risk of harm hoping that the person would die and a murderer who exposed a person to the same risk of harm, but hoped that no injury would occur? And what of the murderer who exposed a person to risk of harm, and simply did not care whether the person was injured or not? The latter depiction is closest to that made by Judge Banks above. He convicted the defendants of murder—murder by indifference.

Conclusion

Despite the success of Cook County prosecutors in the Film Recovery case, prosecuting crimes against health and safety under conventional criminal laws, such as homicide statutes, remains a rare event with doubtful prospects for success. The application of conventional statutes to behavior affecting health and safety is still a legal gamble in a very high stakes game. Although it can be argued that the criminal law serves as an added deterrent, relative to other available civil remedies, it is not clear whether the extra deterrent effect is proportional to the tremendous costs of prosecuting such cases. The more important effect is moral and symbolic. These symbolic values are not as clearly communicated through modern, specialized laws that deal with health and safety problems in technical terms. Though criminal penalties may attach to many of these specialized crimes against health and safety, the stigma associated with those charges is not the same as the stigma that attaches to a conviction for manslaughter, murder, or reckless homicide.

Additional Readings

Berman, Daniel L. *Death on the Job.* New York: Monthly Review Press, 1978.

Bernstein, Dennis and Connie Blitt. "Lethal Dose." *The Progressive* 50 (March 1986): 22–25.

Bollier, David and Joan Claybrook. *Freedom from Harm: The Civilizing Influence of Health, Safety, and Environmental Regulation.* Washington, D.C. and New York: The Public Citizen and Democracy Project, 1986.

Braithwaite, John. *To Punish or Persuade: Enforcement of Coal Mine Safety.* Albany: State University of New York Press, 1985.

Brodeur, Paul. *Outrageous Misconduct: The Asbestos Industry on Trial.* New York: Pantheon, 1985.

Claybrook, Joan and the Staff of Public Citizen. *Retreat From Safety: Reagan's Attack on America's Health.* New York: Pantheon, 1984.

Epstein, Samuel S. *The Politics of Cancer.* San Francisco: Sierra Club Books, 1978.

Ermann, M. David and Richard J. Ludman. "Deviance Against Employees," chap. 4 in *Corporate Deviance.* New York: Holt, Rinehart and Winston, 1982.

Green, Mark and Norman Waitzman. *Business War on the Law: An Analysis of the Benefits of Federal Health/Safety Enforcement,* rev. 2d ed. Washington, D.C.: The Corporate Accountability Research Group, 1981.

McCaffrey, David P. *OSHA and the Politics of Health Regulation.* New York: Plenum, 1982.

Nelkin, Dorothy and Michael S. Brown. *Workers at Risk: Voices from the Workplace.* Chicago: University of Chicago Press, 1984.

Rashke, Richard. *The Killing of Karen Silkwood: The Story Behind the Kerr-McGee Plutonium Case.* Boston: Houghton Mifflin, 1981.

Reasons, Charles E., Lois L. Ross, and Craig Patterson. *Assault on the Worker: Occupational Health and Safety in Canada.* Toronto: Butterworths, 1981.

Scott, Rachel. *Muscle and Blood.* New York: E.P. Dutton, 1974.

Tolchin, Susan J. and Martin Tolchin. *Dismantling America: The Rush to Deregulate.* Boston: Houghton Mifflin, 1983.

Wilson, Graham K. *The Politics of Safety and Health.* New York: Oxford University Press, 1985.

Part III

The Destruction of Community and Environment

Love Canal has become a national symbol for the reckless pollution of the environment that endangers not only the health and safety of individual residents but threatens the very existence of other neighborhoods and communities as well. New York's Love Canal is not the only community that the Hooker and Occidental Chemical companies have threatened with their waste disposal practices. In the article "Chemical Dumping as a Corporate Way of Life," author Matt Tallmer describes a pattern in several states of illegal dumping of chemicals, some perhaps powerful carcinogens: e.g. mirex, a pesticide linked to cancer; and dioxin, the most toxic synthetic compound ever produced. From chemically induced sterility in workers to the poisoning of lake fish and water supplies suspected of causing cancer, bone disease, and birth defects, Tallmer describes the cover-ups and callous attitude of Hooker and Occidental officials toward their dumping practices, which are creating fear and anger in communities in various parts of the country.

The Allied Chemical Company was convicted and fined for its role in the illegal dumping of the highly toxic pesticide Kepone in the James River in Virginia. As the level of Kepone in oysters and fish increased, the Governor finally closed about 100 miles of the river, which virtually destroyed the fishing industry for two years in the region. Allied Chemical did bear the costs of burying the contaminated plant and surrounding topsoil. The problems created by this illegal dumping of Kepone have cost the Environmental Protection Agency millions of dollars, and there are thousands of pounds of this toxic chemical still precariously lying on the riverbed. In addition, numerous employees exposed to this dangerous pesticide experienced severe tremors, liver and brain damage, personality changes, diminished ability to walk and stand, and signs of sterility. Even some

109

of the family members of the workers were affected through Kepone traces that showed up in laundered clothes.

Yet as Christopher Stone asks in his article "A Slap on the Wrist for the Kepone Mob," who really pays the price for this catastrophe? No one has gone to jail for poisoning Virginia's environment and damaging the health of the chemical plant workers. And despite evidence of the company's attempt to cover up what should be defined as "criminal" actions, none of Allied Chemical's officials have been fined or punished. In the aftermath of this disaster, Stone discusses the limits of the criminal justice system in pinpointing individual responsibility and controlling the injurious actions of large impersonal corporations. Stone, a university law professor, proposes some innovative legal reforms to restructure the internal organization of convicted corporations that might help prevent future environmental disasters.

In the last article in this section, "Who's Burning Boston?," James Brady, a sociologist and Director of the Arson Task Force in the city of Boston, provides a trenchant analysis of one of the most destructive and fastest growing crimes in America: arson for profit. Brady challenges the popular stereotypes of arsonists as simply pathological pyromaniacs, vandals, or persons with personal grudges. Frequently, the author contends, arson involves a vast network of corrupt officials in police and fire departments, insurance company personnel, professional "torches," and organized criminal racketeers. But as Brady argues, the greatest profits accrue to respectable banks and real estate corporations whose lending policies and development practices, such as "redlining," "blockbusting," and land speculation in transitional neighborhoods, create the incentives for arson. The victims, however, are not only those persons burned to death or driven from their homes or small shops, but entire communities transformed into "urban deserts" or "gentrified" islands of luxury apartments and condominiums inaccessible to the burned out tenants.

9 / Chemical Dumping as a Corporate Way of Life

MATT TALLMER

If you head south for ninety miles or so from Sacramento, California, you get to Lathrop, a town of about 2,000 people—too small to have its own newspaper. What Lathrop does have is a chemical plant operated by the Occidental Chemical Company. Oxy, as the company is called, is owned by the Hooker Chemical and Plastics Company of Buffalo, New York. Hooker, in turn, is a subsidiary of Occidental Petroleum. People in Lathrop admit that if it weren't for the chemical plant, the town would not appear on the map. The people would have nowhere to work.

Michael Trout lived in Lathrop for most of his life. After he got married, he applied for a job at *the* local business—Oxy. The only job open was on the night shift, but Trout took it. He needed work. That was in 1970.

Trout began his term at Oxy by cleaning up the barrels and drums that day-shift workers would leave lying around the plant. Four years later, he was transferred to the Agriculture Chemical Division, where pesticides were made and stored. One of the pesticides Trout worked with was DBCP, which is suspected of causing cancer, birth defects, and male sterility.

Barely a year after the transfer, Trout began having dizzy spells. Then he began to feel nauseated, and then came migraine headaches. He went to his family doctors but they could find nothing wrong. Finally, one doctor sent him the ninety miles north to see a specialist in Sacramento. The doctor found that Trout had brain cancer. In February 1976, Trout underwent an operation to remove the tumors. After several months at home, his headaches, dizziness, and nausea stopped, and he went back to work.

But during his absence, workers at the plant had begun talking among themselves about his cancer and about the illnesses that were affecting many of them. They went to the company and demanded

111

that Hooker start testing the workers. The tests found Trout and twenty-seven of his fellow workers to be sterile.

The twenty-eight workers filed suit against Hooker and Oxy, charging that their sterility had been caused by the chemicals they worked with and, in some cases, made. But they all kept working at the plant. It was the only business in town. Trout went to a company official and told him of his cancer, and his suspicion that it was caused by chemicals. The executive told Trout he had to prove it in order to get the company to do anything. Trout had no proof, and did not know how to begin to get it, so he let the matter drop.

In December 1979, Trout started having migraines again. Then came the nausea and the dizzy spells. He knew what it was. After an operation to remove this cancer, he died on December 15, at the age of twenty-eight.

In March 1980, his widow, Marta Trout, filed a $4.5 million wrongful death suit against Oxy and Hooker. "I am charging," she said, "that he died as a result of chemical exposures. That type of tumor is showing up in chemical workers throughout the country." Hooker denied that charge in court papers, but a year after the suit was filed *The New York Times* printed an article showing that chemical workers were, indeed, coming down with the same type of tumor.

Marta Trout is not the only widow of an Oxy worker to file suit. In 1979, Barbara Allen filed suit against the company charging that her late husband, William, had died as a result of exposure to the pesticide DBCP. "We have evidence that Hooker officials knew that if DBCP was improperly handled it caused cancer and sterility," said Robert Ciaetti, Barbara Allen's attorney. "The company provided no warning to the workers, no protective equipment, nothing."

Another Hooker employee at Lathrop has also filed suit, charging that his son's birth defects were caused by DBCP.

Shortly after Michael Trout died and the lawsuits started at Lathrop, the Environmental Protection Agency banned DBCP in forty-eight states—all but Alaska and Hawaii. But that did not stop Hooker officials from writing a two-page memo discussing the possibility of re-entering the DBCP market, should the ban be lifted. The memo, on Hooker stationery, lists six mathematical steps to determine whether risk to the company is low enough. Among them:

- "Determine the normal temporary or permanent sterility rate in the general population. Also the normal cancer rate for the type of tumor DBCP is suspected of causing."
- "Assume that 50 percent of the normal rate for those exposed may file claims; determine the number of potential claims for cancer and sterility."

• "Estimate the probable average judgment or settlement which would result from a claim; calculate the potential liability."

The memo concluded that there was no "significant risk due to exposures at the planned levels." What risk there was, one Hooker document noted, boiled down to "the potential economic impact of litigation by people who might claim to be affected."

Hooker Chemical's corporate reputation was, of course, seriously tarnished by the international media attention focused on Love Canal, the site of an old company waste dump. Love Canal got its name from civil engineer William T. Love, who dreamed of building a canal around nearby Niagara Falls in the late 1880s. The plan fell through after a depression cut off all of Love's money, and in the late 1930s the site was sold to Hooker, which used the abandoned canal as a dump site for hundreds of tons of chemicals and chemical wastes. In 1953 Hooker turned the land over to the local school board. The school board sold it to a private developer who built houses on top of the chemical barrels. A generation later, as leaching wastes began to be linked to miscarriages, birth defects, and other ailments, more than 200 families fled their homes.

Most people assume that Love Canal is the only place where Hooker left its dirty footprints. They are wrong. One Congressional staff member who has investigated chemical waste disposal, but did not want his name used, said, "Hooker is one of the handful of companies that do this again and again. When we caught one of the big boys—the DuPonts or Dows—doing it, they cleaned it up, paid for health studies, and provided money to study the pollution effects. Hooker fights you every step of the way."

Niagara Falls, New York, like Lathrop, California, is a small town that has provided several episodes in the long history of mishaps at Hooker facilities.

In December 1975, a tank car on the grounds of Hooker's chemical plant in Niagara Falls exploded, spewing over several miles its toxic payload—chlorine gas, which was used as a chemical warfare agent during World War I. Four Hooker workers died in the accident, and eighty others were hospitalized, including five people who had been in a department store five miles away from the blast. Two workers died in a 1960 accident that exposed them to another toxic gas. More recently, reports have surfaced suggesting that workers at the Niagara Falls plant have been regularly exposed to dioxin. An epidemiological study by the Oil, Chemical, and Atomic Workers Union shows unusually high rates of lung, liver, and kidney cancer, leukemia rates almost triple the average, and increased rates of birth defects, spontaneous abortions, miscarriages, and stillbirths among the workers' families.

Also in Niagara Falls, across town from the Love Canal neighborhood, is a forested area with a bird sanctuary and a creek. Because of the creek's deep red clay base, it is known as Bloody Run Creek. Indians who once lived on its banks believed it ran with blood, not water. Just off its banks stands the two-level, wood frame house of Fred Armagost. His son Wayne, and Wayne's family, used to live there. As a boy Wayne swam and fished in the creek; his three young children used to do the same.

In 1978, Wayne Armagost lost his job because he had "chronic breathing problems." At times, he simply could not breathe properly. His children all suffer from similarly mysterious symptoms. The entire family has been through a battery of medical tests, but none of the examinations has pinpointed the cause of their illnesses. But the Armagosts, and a pediatrician from the New York State Department of Health, think they know what caused them. They believe they are suffering because of Bloody Run Creek. And, says Fred Armagost, the Department of Health doctor has seen an improvement in Wayne's children since they moved away from it.

Starting in the early 1950s, just after the dump at Love Canal closed, Hooker began dumping chemicals into a ditch on the banks of Bloody Run Creek. At the last count, there were more than 80,000 tons of chemical wastes there. In 1979, the New York State Department of Environmental Conservation issued a report on toxic wastes in New York State. The Department charged that the Bloody Run Creek dump was "run rather carelessly by Hooker." The drums were thrown into an open-air pit, and Hooker officials at the scene made little attempt to cover them with dirt. As a result, large quantities of chemicals have leached off the site, contaminating the surrounding area and the creek.

Hooker dumped a variety of chemicals into the pit, including benzene, which has been called the most powerful carcinogen known; Mirex, a pesticide linked to cancer and sterility; dioxin, the most toxic synthetic compound ever made, and 2,4,5-Trichlorophenol, a pesticide used in making Agent Orange, the Vietnam defoliant.

In 1976, the Environmental Protection Agency took soil samples in and around the dump. Mirex was found at levels of seventy-nine parts per million a few hundred yards away from the site, but on the site itself, the levels were found only in the parts per billion. The EPA's safe level of Mirex is 0.9 parts per billion.

But even more upsetting to area residents and environmental experts are the reports of water pollution. As in most rural areas, the Niagara Falls residents get their drinking water from underground wells, which tap the groundwater supply in the aquifers. The state Department of Environmental Conservation reported that there is "likely contamination of the area's groundwaters." Water samples taken by both the EPA and the state show dangerously high levels of Mirex, benzene, and 2,4,5-Trichlorophenol. "If that's true," one EPA official said, "then the residents have been drinking that crap for years. All we can do is sit back and watch the cancers develop."

At the other end of New York state, just sixty miles east of New York City and five stops away on the Long Island Railroad, is the town of Hicksville. It has all the ingredients of a typical Long Island suburb: one private school, appropriately named Hicksville High, a volunteer fire department, no local police force, no hospital—nothing to distinguish it from the myriad of other Nassau County suburbs that sprang up just after World War II.

Except the chemical plant. Since 1947, Hooker has operated a facility on New South Road in Hicksville. Before Hooker took it over, the plant was used to make rubber during the war. Under Hooker, the plant has made a polyvinyl chloride, a plastic used in most of the plastic products on the market. When polyvinyl chloride (pvc) is made, the process produces waste forms of pvc, vinyl chloride (vc), and vc monomer—a carcinogenic gas. Both pvc and vc cause angiosarcoma of the liver, until recently the rarest form of cancer known. They also cause acro-osteolysis, a degenerative disease of the bones in the hand and fingers; over a period of years the bones become so brittle they snap under the slightest pressure.

Hooker was well aware of acro-osteolysis and its causes; through the Chemical Manufacturers Association, it helped sponsor the 1973 research at the University of Michigan which pinpointed the disease. The chemical firm was also aware of a New York State law, Article 27 of the Environmental Conservation Law, which forbids the dumping of hazardous wastes without a permit. Hooker had no permit to dump on Long Island.

In 1977 the Department of Environmental Conservation sent a hazardous waste survey to all chemical companies in the state. The document, to be filled out by a state official with information provided by the company, listed what wastes were produced by each plant, and where they were being disposed of. Hooker told an official from the Department that the Hicksville plant wastes were being shipped to "unknown . . . off-site dumps" in New Jersey. Two years later, it became apparent that Hooker's response did not correspond with the facts.

In June 1979, a House subcommittee investigating hazardous waste disposal released a Hooker memo which reported that from 1946 until 1968 "any and all solid wastes in drums" from the Hicksville plant were shipped to an old municipal landfill in the nearby town of Syosset, in clear violation of Article 27. The barrels contained vc, pvc, vc resin, and TMA, a chemical which causes inflammation of the lungs and short-circuits the body's immunological system. After that dump was shut down, the wastes were shipped to another municipal dump in Bethpage, to the southeast of Hicksville. There, in addition to the chemicals and wastes dumped at Syosset, the company dumped DMF, a highly toxic acid, and "various other organic residues." Hooker also sent to the Bethpage landfill drums that were too damaged to be resold. The entire project was a fiasco for the company: As of 1978 there were 478,300 pounds of what Hooker memos called "major current environmental pollution" at the dump. Workers had been sprayed with liquid wastes, and once a truck left a half-mile trail of wastes along a public street.

In 1973, the operators of the Bethpage dump refused to take any more barrels and drums from Hooker. The truckloads "smelled bad" and created "problems." Memos released by the Congressional subcommittee indicated Hooker's uncertainty about where its own wastes were going. They said the firm shipped the wastes to a "private (?) landfill in Brentwood." There is only one landfill in Brentwood, and no traces of vc-related chemicals have been found in it. But in April 1980, vc monomer *was* found in a school in Hauppauge, two miles from Brentwood. The substance was found to be coming from a landfill in that town, next door to the school. Hooker is the only producer of vc in any form on Long Island, and Nassau County health chief Dr. David Harris blamed the presence of the chemical in the school on the company—a charge that Hooker denies.

Before the apparent dumping began at Bethpage and Hauppauge, two in-house solutions to the growing pollution problem were turned down. A suggestion to build a plasticizer recovery plant at Hicksville was rejected as "not economically attractive," and an idea to build an incinerator was turned down because "the capital costs would be high."

The Bethpage landfill is virtually next door to Grumman Aerospace's huge plant. Today, two Grumman wells have been closed because traces of vc or pvc have been found in them. "We believe Grumman workers have been drinking contaminated water for years," said Donald Middleton, the head of the Long Island office of the State Department of Environmental Conservation, "contaminated because of Hooker's dumping." Grumman officials discovered the contamination in 1973 and first went to Hooker and asked that the company clean up its mess. When Hooker refused to answer Grumman's letters, the company sent its evidence against Hooker to the Department of Environmental Conservation. The Department quickly hauled Hooker officials into a private meeting, so that executives of the chemical firm could explain the situation. According to confidential notes of the meeting, "A representative of Hooker stated inasmuch as Hooker was the only producer of vc in the area, the company would accept responsibility for vc in the Grumman wells." When Hooker officials publicly denied responsibility, the state slapped Hooker with a fine of more than $500,000.

In tiny Taft, Louisiana, Hooker has another chemical plant. Many farmers in the surrounding communities have complained for years that the smoke belching from the plant's stacks was killing their crops and livestock. But it was not until last year that state and Federal investigators began looking at the plant's operations. One state investigator conceded that "we really don't know what all the facts are. [But there] are definitely some problems down there."

The agencies are looking into charges that Hooker conducted an open-air dumping operation, similar to the one at Bloody Run Creek and possibly with the same results. "The problem," said former Federal investigator Gary Keyser, "is that they just threw the stuff out into the air and let it rot."

Dumping has not been the least of Louisiana's chemical problems. In 1974, 140 private contractors hired to build an addition to a Hooker plant in the state sued the company, charging that exposures to chlorine have left them impotent, sterile, and without the senses of taste and smell. All the cases were settled out of court, for amounts ranging from $7,000 to $250,000, after a physician hired by Hooker wound up backing the contractor's claims. Dr. Robert Henkin, a Georgetown University specialist in taste and smell, said he was worried about the builders' possible exposure to a cancer-causing agent.

"Another of my concerns," Henkin said, "is that there were no follow-up studies. The company wanted to know what was wrong with them, so they could settle the case, but they showed no concern by simply following up on these men, to see what the long-term effects were." Five of the workers have since died.

Fifty miles west of Jacksonville, Florida, Hooker runs a phosphate processing plant in the town of White Springs. The plant is on the banks of the Suwanee River, which environmental officials believed was one of the last unpolluted rivers in the United States. Now they aren't sure.

In 1978, the Florida Department of Environmental Regulation began receiving reports of possible air and water emissions violations by Hooker. In June 1979, the Department found that Hooker had written a facility assessment report on the White Springs plant three months earlier. Officials requested a copy of the report and Hooker refused. After a brief skirmish in court, Hooker agreed to give them an edited copy of the report. That version contained enough evidence to make Hooker and three company executives plead no contest to charges of violating the emissions standards and attempting to cover up the violations.

The legal limit on fluoride emissions into the air amounts to thirty-four pounds per day at White Springs. "The document proved the plant couldn't meet our rules," said John Bottcher, assistant counsel for the Department of Environmental Regulation. But "for economic reasons," Hooker's own report noted, the plant continued to give off 400 pounds of fluoride daily—except when the Department of Environmental Regulation tested the air, when it switched to a cleaner but less profitable chemical mix. Hooker never told this to the Department.

The company also kept two sets of air emissions test results. The reports which showed the plant operating in compliance with the rules were given to the state investigators. The others were hidden in company files. The assessment report also informed state officials that "it was necessary to retest the plant five or six times" to get a test showing compliance.

Residents of the area have known for years that Hooker discharged plant wastes directly into the Suwanee River. Department of Environmental Regulation investigators have subpoenaed and received the edited portions of the assessment report in an attempt to "shed some light" on the discharges.

In 1977, a former employe at Hooker's White Lake, Michigan, plant started talking to the state environmental officials. The officials had long suspected that something was wrong at the plant because scores of dead fish would wash up after Hooker had "disposed of" chemicals. Now they believed they knew what the trouble was: Hooker, the former employe said, was taking barrels of chemical waste and dumping them on vacant company property behind the plant. When confronted with these charges, Hooker executives merely said that they had "a few—maybe twenty or thirty" barrels behind the plant. James Truchan, the supervisor of environmental enforcement, showed up at the plant one afternoon. He found more than 20,000 barrels. "Hooker just took the stuff and dumped it wherever the hell they damn well pleased," Truchan said.

Two years after the dump was discovered, the state of Michigan took the company to court; Hooker executives had been "less than cooperative" about cleaning it up, the state charged. The company settled out of court and agreed to pay for clean-up (estimated at close to $20 million) and pay more than $1 million in penalties. In addition,

Occidental posted a $2 million guarantee on the clean-up in case Hooker did not fulfill its obligations. Three summers ago, state officials warned area residents against drinking the water or eating fish from White Lake. The water contained dangerous amounts of Mirex, dioxin, and Kepone, one of the most toxic chemicals. Area residents say they have increased rates of birth defects, cancer, sterility, heart attacks, convulsions, and nerve damage. The state has been looking into that. In June 1980, a Federal grand jury was empaneled by U.S. Attorney James Brady to look into charges that Hooker officials had covered up the dumpings for more than twenty years. It was later dismissed with no action taken. Truchan says now "our concerns are with clean-up."

Back in Lathrop, California, a document surfaced two years ago that sheds new light on the Occidental Chemical Company's operations in that little town. The document was a memo from a safety engineer to his boss. "I really don't feel comfortable signing this," he wrote. "However, I don't feel it would be wise to explain the discrepancy to the state at this time." The discrepancy concerned the disposal of "Oxy's" wastes. Oxy had told the California authorities the wastes were being "processed" and shipped, by truck, around the country. The truth was that Oxy had been burying the wastes behind the plant since 1953.

The company dumped DDT, DEF (another deadly pesticide), DBCP, uranium, and radium in its own back yard. Tools found in the pits were so "hot" from radiation that they were taken to a high-level dump site for reburial. One Oxy executive wrote to another that if "we stop [dumping] now, we may escape unnoticed."

Other Oxy memos noted that the dumping had "destroyed the usability of several area wells." Wells near the dump site were "contaminated to the point of being poisonous to animals and possibly to humans," one memo noted. One neighbor told Federal investigators that his dog had died after drinking well water, and that he had become quite sick. Yet Oxy went right on dumping, until state authorities caught up with the company two years ago. Oxy and Hooker now face fines of $25,000 per day, per violation.

So far, the Hooker Chemical and Plastics Company and the Occidental Chemical Company have been hauled into court in Florida, Michigan, California, and New York (in a civil, not criminal, prosecution). The states of Louisiana, New Jersey, New York, and Ohio are now investigating Hooker or Oxy operations. Many more states would join the ranks, if they took the advice of James Truchan of Michigan, who spent four years investigating Hooker operations at White Lake. He took the company to court and got it to pay for the wasteland it had created. "Any state which has a Hooker plant in it had better take a damn good, long, hard look at that plant," Truchan said. "They have no regard for anything but getting rid of their wastes, and they don't care where they put it or what they do with it."

But long, hard looks won't help Michael Trout. Or William Allen. Or Wayne Armatgost.

10 / A Slap on the Wrist for the Kepone Mob

CHRISTOPHER D. STONE

As more activities in our society are taken over by large-scale organizations, an increasing share of misconduct will originate in the corporate sector. This puts our legal system to a test. When the wrongdoer is a corporation, or employees hidden in the shadows of a vast bureaucratic latticework, are our present rules and institutions adequate? Can they daunt companies into setting up the appropriate organizational machinery—the quality control systems and the ways to monitor compliance with the law? Can the rules penetrate to the worker level and stay the hand of an employee who finds himself at the edge of a reckless act? These are large and important questions, whose answers, in the aftermath of the Kepone affair, are worrying.

Background

In 1950, scientists working at Allied Chemical came up with an insecticide related to DDT, but apparently more effective against DDT-resistant organisms and quite likely even more persistent in the environment. Allied originally licensed Kepone production to others, but in 1966, as demand grew, it began manufacture in its own plant in Hopewell, Virginia.

A highly toxic pesticide, Kepone is not a product whose dangers should have caught anyone off guard. Indeed, several studies, including one by Allied itself in the early 1960s, had already noted the tendency of the compound to induce "DDT-like tremors." Tests on rats showed kidney lesions in females and atrophy of the testes in males. Liver abnormalities—including enlargement, "congestion," and lesions—suggested a possible cancer link. Other researchers noted "whole-body tremor" and liver enlargement in quail. Studies on hens and mice revealed impaired reproductive performance, even among the offspring of test animals.

But commercial production continued unabated.

121

Then, in the spring of 1973, amid circumstances that have inspired some skepticism, Allied decided to move Kepone production out of its Hopewell facility. The explanation the company eventually offered the courts and congressional committees was that it needed the floor space for expanded production of other products. The Hopewell plant was under the direction of the chemical division. Kepone was a product of the agricultural division. Thus, if something really had to go, there was a certain organizational logic to pushing Kepone out.

Kepone went, but not very far—next door, to be precise, into an abandoned gasoline filling station. This odd new home was not leased (as it might undoubtedly have been) by Allied itself, but by a new Virginia corporation set up for no other purpose than to process Kepone exclusively for Allied.

The new outfit, ironically named Life Science Products, Inc., had two stockholders, William Moore and Virgil Hundtofte, both former employees of Allied. Each put into the company perhaps $500 or $1,000 of his own money (their testimony varied). On top of this modest equity cushion, however, a Richmond bank was willing to make them a $175,000 loan. Nominally, Life Science Products was the borrower. But in fact, Allied agreed with LSP to make the repayments through a "surcharge" Allied would pay on each pound of Kepone, until the loan had been retired.

Other provisions of Allied's contract with LSP give evidence that the risks did not go uncontemplated. One clause provides for LSP to indemnify Allied against any kind of liability arising from the production process. Another contemplates that in the event any environmental rulings should halt production, the parties would confer about bringing the plant into compliance. If modifications were feasible, LSP was to make them, but in point of economic fact, Allied would again pay through a "surcharge."

Production of Kepone began in the converted gasoline station in March 1974, under conditions that almost defy description. Brian Kelly, in his *Washington Star* series on the Kepone affair, reported

an incredible mess. Dust flying through the air . . . saturating the workers' clothing, getting into their hair, even into sandwiches they munched in production areas.

The Kepone dust sometimes blew . . . in clouds. A gas station operator across the street said it obscured his view of the Life Science Plant. . . . Two firemen in a station behind Life Science say there were times when they wondered if they could see well enough to wheel their engines out in response to a fire alarm.

Workers at LSP began to develop the "Kepone shakes," sometimes within two weeks of starting work. Turnover was high. By April, the sewage digesters in Hopewell's municipal sewage treatment plant began malfunctioning; the Kepone was killing the bacteria on which the sewage digestion process depended.

The undoing of LSP seems troublingly fortuitous but, once in motion, swift. Local doctors who had examined some of the workers, ordinarily on the basis of "informal agreements" with the company, diagnosed their problems as "hypertension" or the like, and prescribed tranquilizers or psychotherapy. But in July 1975, one of the workers had become skeptical and found his way into the office of a young independent internist from Taiwan, who, baffled by the symptoms, sent blood and urine samples to the Center for Disease Control (CDC) in Atlanta. At CDC, the blood was discovered to be so high in Kepone that the toxicologists suspected the sample had been contaminated through mishandling. Nevertheless they notified the state epidemiologist, just in case he wanted to pursue the matter. That was on a Friday.

By Monday morning the epidemiologist, Dr. Robert Jackson, had verified the serious condition of the sample donor by phone. On Wednesday he began personally to examine workers as they came off the day shift.

> The first man I saw was a 23-year-old who was so sick he was unable to stand due to unsteadiness, was suffering severe chest pains . . . had severe tremor, abnormal eye movements, was disoriented.

Jackson immediately arranged for the worker to be admitted to the hospital, and he proceeded to review a parade of similar symptoms as each of the other workers came in.

On Thursday, July 24, 1975, LSP's operations were brought to a close.

What was the Toll?

In cases of this sort, there can never be a consensus on the final costs. On some of the damages it is hard to place a value, and as for others, only time will tell. The first 133 workers tested *all* had traces of Kepone in their blood, and over half had symptoms of clinical illness. In addition to severe tremors, their problems included weight loss, liver tenderness and enlargement, brain damage, chest pains, personality changes, eye flutters, and diminished ability to walk or stand. At least fourteen showed signs of sterility. Some of the employees' family members were affected as well, apparently through Kepone traces in the household wash.

The workers' problems having drawn wide-spread attention, an investigation was made of Kepone's effects in the environment. Significant quantities of Kepone dust were found to have ranged from the plant at least sixteen miles in the air and sixty-four miles in the water. Forty people who did not work at LSP but lived in the vicinity of the plant showed traces of Kepone in their blood, although at considerably lower levels than LSP employees. The National Cancer Institute undertook a study which reinforced earlier suspicions that Kepone could induce liver cancer (although Allied's recent studies indicate otherwise). An examination of frozen seafood taken from the historic James River below Hopewell—a major fishing and shellfishing region—showed that Kepone had been appearing in oysters since 1968, and in fish no later than 1970. In December 1975, Governor Mills E. Godwin, Jr., closed approximately 100 miles of the James to all fishing, pending further analysis.

Most, perhaps all, fishing has since been reallowed, partly as a result of cleanup, partly as a result of upward revisions in the ever-controversial Kepone "action level." Meanwhile, the loss to fishing and allied industries has been estimated to range from $4 million to $24 million. Some of the cleanup costs, including burning and burying the plant and adjacent topsoil, were borne by Allied. But EPA has spent an additional $3.5 million. Disposal of the remaining wastes, much of which is still in storage, will run into millions more. Some people are worried about the thousands of pounds of Kepone that still lie on the riverbed, but total removal would cost anywhere from $100 to $500 million, and, when all the dredging was done, might disrupt the environment more than removal of the poison would be worth.

Various criminal charges were lodged against Allied and LSP officials. Allied, it turned out, had not duly reported, and allegedly had taken steps to conceal, its dumping of Kepone into the Gravelly Run, a tributary of the James, during the years 1966–1974, when production was carried out in its own plant. For this, Virgil Hundtofte and four other men working at the time for Allied were charged with conspiracy to defraud the United States. Hundtofte was allowed to plead guilty to a misdemeanor in return for agreeing to turn state's evidence against the other four, two of whom thereupon pleaded guilty. The remaining defendants—the Allied plant's two top officers—demanded trial. They claimed that the unreported discharges were intended to be only intermittent and temporary, and they were ultimately acquitted. U. S. District Judge Robert R. Merhige, Jr., explained, "I simply am not satisfied beyond a reasonable doubt. It is as simple as that." After this turn of events, the prosecution felt it unfair to hang the entire rap on the subordinates, and their charges were also dismissed, even though they had pleaded guilty.

Thus, when all was said and done, no individual was held accountable for all the years in which Allied was somehow—impersonally, one presumes—violating the law.

As top-level employees of LSP, Moore and Hundtofte faced deeper problems from actions arising during the period of LSP's production. They were charged with 153 counts of violating the federal Water Pollution Control Act, charges on which each might have been fined $3.8 million. Both men pleaded no contest and were fined $25,000 and placed on five years' probation. One of them is reportedly in retirement, while the other has become manager of a fertilizer plant in New Mexico.

The corporate defendants have had a mixed fate. Life Science Products, all but defunct by the time of trial, was convicted and "fined" $3.8 million for 153 violations of the Water Pollution Control Act. This vindicated the law's bark, perhaps, but there turned out to be nothing left in the cupboard to bite.

Allied, by contrast, had the wherewithal to make good on a judgment, but establishing its liability was more complex. At the start the prosecution wanted to hold Allied responsible for the crimes of LSP. Under the legal doctrine called "piercing the corporate veil," a court may, under certain circumstances, hold a parent corporation jointly liable with a subsidiary company for the commission of wrong acts by the subsidiary. The approach makes things easier for the prosecution, because it allows conviction of the parent without having to prove its actual participation or knowledge—much as the wrongs of an agent will, in ordinary circumstances, simply be imputed to his principal, whether or not the principal can be shown to have known the details.

LSP, however, had been established not as a technical subsidiary, with Allied owning all or substantially all of its stock, but as "an independent contractor," however thinly capitalized and pseudo-separate its existence. This forced the government to charge that Allied "aided and abetted" LSP in its wrongs. In order to prove this accusation the government had to prove, at the very least, that Allied had actual knowledge of LSP's wrongdoings. Because of the burden of proof requirement in criminal cases, this is difficult to show. Allied was acquitted on the basis of "insufficient evidence."

Allied did not get off so easily for the pollution which occurred before it moved the Kepone production out of its own plant. The company pleaded no contest to 940 counts of violating federal water pollution control laws from 1971 through 1974. Judge Merhige (perhaps skeptical, in the back of his mind, about the relationship with LSP) fined the company the maximum of each count, $13.24 million in all. This was the largest criminal fine ever levied in an environmental suit.

But having exacted this enormous fine, Judge Merhige at once proceeded to air his own misgivings. He realized that such a fine would pass into general federal revenues, with nothing earmarked for the people of Virginia, who had been hurt most. The judge therefore suggested that if Allied should take voluntary measures "to alleviate the horrendous effects that have occurred" in Virginia, his mind would not be closed "to consideration of an appropriate" reduction of the fine.

Allied quickly agreed to donate $8 million to a nonprofit corporation, the Virginia Environmental Endowment. In the words of Allied's attorney, the new corporation would "fund scientific research projects and implement remedial projects and other programs to help alleviate the problem that Kepone has created . . . and . . . enhance and improve the overall quality of the environment in Virginia. . . ." In view of the amount of the donation as well as the cleanup costs Allied had borne, plus a contribution the company had made to fund Kepone-related medical research, the court reduced the originally announced $13.24 million fine to $5 million.

From the corporation's point of view, this action involved more than just changing the names of some checks. Income tax laws do not allow a company to treat *criminal fines* as a tax-deductible cost of doing business. The company has, however, claimed the *donation* as a goodwill expense, reducing the true after-tax costs by approximately $4 million. Allied must also have hoped, at least originally, that to the extent the endowment's disbursements mitigated the injuries Kepone caused, the money would do double service, reducing the claims that could be made in civil suits by those who were partly compensated out of the fund. (The U. S. Attorney, William B. Cummings, has foreseen that angle. He claims that the court-appointed directors of the endowment, including himself, are determined to avoid allowing a fine, which was originally intended to be a deterrent, to offset the civil liability imposed by law. If the directors pursue this course, the endowment, just now beginning operation, will be in the ironic position of repairing environmental damage in Virginia caused by anything *but* Kepone.)

The third corporation to be charged was the city of Hopewell, whose prosecution also raised questions of national significance. Most critics of corporate behavior have focused their attention on business corporations, while their venerable cousins, the municipal corporations, have by and large escaped the heat. Not that municipal corporations are better citizens. The Environmental Protection Agency has complained that while 90 percent of major industries are expected to meet the 1977 water discharge targets, only half the cities and towns are living up to their schedules. And whatever knowledge Allied's top management actually had, there can be no doubt that Hopewell officials knew of LSP's Kepone discharges no later than the breakdown of the municipal sewage plant, two months after production began. Yet the city—which proclaims itself "Chemical Capital of the South" (meaning its annual city budget of about $12 million comes largely from its chemical company constituents, of which Allied is the largest)—did nothing but seek quiet accommodations.

Such cozy arrangements, in which cities wink at or abet the overburdening of their sewage facilities, have been all too common. Thus, according to *Business Week*, EPA officials were particularly anxious for the government to take a tough stance against Hopewell, which faced $3.9 million in fines. The judgment: The city was let off with $10,000 and five years' probation.

What Good Did the Law Do?

In retrospect, what judgments can one make about the adequacy of the social system to prevent such criminal indifference in the future? The primary issue, certainly, is that raised by Judge Merhige in handing down the judgments.

> I hope after this sentence, that every corporate official, every corporate employee that has reason to think that pollution is going on, will think, "If I don't do something about it now, I am apt to be out of a job tomorrow."

A splendid aim, to be sure. The problem is that such concern will not automatically reverberate through the company just because the corporate controller, off in headquarters, has been forced to write a check to the U. S. Treasury. There will be fundamental changes in attitude only when the demands of society become moving forces in the employee's environment, where they are now too often subordinate to other claims: the judgment of peers, the demands and expectations of superiors. The law, for its part, can penetrate this corporate culture only if its threats are brought home to the worker. This can happen either directly, through the imposition of penalties, or indirectly, through forcing top management (against all the weight of institutional inertia) to alter the reward and incentive scheme of the organization.

In the Kepone affair, no one went to prison. Not a single employee of Allied was fined. None, so far as is known, lost his or her job, was passed over for promotion, or suffered censure from any of the professional societies that might have exercised some voice in the matter.

Moore and Hundtofte, it is true, have suffered substantial fines for their role at Life Science Products. But it must be remembered that they were sole shareholders and top officers in a very small corporation. There simply was not enough bureaucratic and physical distance between themselves and the wrongdoing to make their protests of ignorance credible. Thus, their fate, it seems to me, has only limited implication for those who work in giant corporations like Allied, where acocuntability is inevitably too divided and shadowy for any Moores and Hundtoftes to be handy.

As for Allied itself, the total estimated cash outflow connected with the criminal actions (in other words, corrected for the reduction in corporate income tax) was expected to be $9.5 million. But does anyone really suppose that this will force any of Allied's executives to take a cut in compensation? The brunt of the fine is passed through "the corporation" and spread over 28,500,000 shares of stock, as a nonrecurring loss of about 33 cents a share—nothing to toss out management for, even if such uprisings were otherwise feasible.

Myriad civil suits have been filed against Allied, it is true. These include suits on behalf of workers and their families, fishermen, marina owners, the Commonwealth of Virginia, and others; some have already been settled for undisclosed sums. The final figures will almost certainly exceed the payments exacted in the criminal action. Nonetheless, as Allied reported to the Securities and Exchange Commission in a recent filing, it has $101 million worth of insurance, and "it is believed . . . that any loss ultimately sustained . . . will not seriously affect the company's financial position."

None of this is to suggest that the various Kepone judgments, after deduction of coinsurance and taxes, will be unfelt. The whole episode must be an embarrassment to a company that likes to think well of itself (and has many reasons to). But in a corporation with over $2.6 billion in annual sales, there is no guarantee that the internal ramifications will persist except among the public relations cadre.

The Old Shell Game

There are several related issues of considerable significance. The first of these has to do with the old corporate shell game. I am not as much interested in judging Allied's true motives in helping LSP get started as in the interpretation of the judicial outcome by the corporate community. Allied was absolved of liability for the criminal acts of LSP on the grounds that LSP was not, strictly speaking, a subsidiary, but an "independent contractor"—a stalking horse, some think, of more subtle shading. Indeed, had Allied arranged LSP's existence at the start, in 1966, presumably it could have cut off its own criminal liability altogether. If this is the law, what encouragement will it give other companies, contemplating high-risk ventures, to set up similar "suppliers"?

Another set of questions has to do with the uneven treatment of the two types of entities, Hopewell the town and Allied the corporation. On what legal and moral bases should the business's stockholders bear the brunt of a heavy fine, while the municipality's taxpayers go relatively scot free? Judge Merhige said he saw no purpose in doling out heavy fines against Hopewell, since it would amount to nothing more than "a transfer of dollars from one pocket of the taxpayer to another." But surely this is specious: A heavy fine against Hopewell would have redounded to the benefit of taxpayers elsewhere. And there would have been some justice in making Hopewell's residents pay because they had been the direct financial beneficiaries of the city's cutting corners on sewage treatment. Worse, by not treating their sewage adequately, Hopewell's taxpayers had imposed costs on others, including communities downstream, oystermen, and fishermen, whose civil remedies against a municipality are, I suspect, quite limited. Allied's far-flung shareholders knew less, if anything, than a lot of people around Hopewell. And, culpability aside, does anyone really suppose that a heavy fine is more calculated to mobilize political housecleaning among Allied's shareholders than among Hopewell's voters?

If Hopewell's fate was light, the fate of the various public agencies that had a hand in the matter was even lighter. Consider their record:

The Virginia Air Quality Resources Board maintained an air-monitoring filter only a few hundred yards from the LSP plant. Unfortunately, Kepone was not among the list of things the station had been told to check on, and the data the board demanded of the plant required no appraisal of Kepone's toxicity or potentially hazardous nature.

The state Water Quality Control Board realized there was a serious problem of noncompliance during a routine check in October 1974, when it discovered a huge pit filling with Kepone. At that time company and local sewage officials were to deal with the Kepone problem. The board had the authority to close the plant down (one of its people seems to have been so inclined), but decided to try persuasion instead.

The Virginia Department of Labor and Industry might have done something, but federal law preempts states from enforcing their own work-place standards until approved by the federal Occupational Safety and Health Administration, before whom Virginia's plan had been moldering for two years. In autumn 1974, OSHA received a complaint from an LSP employee who claimed to have been fired for refusal to work under unsafe conditions. OSHA's response was merely to write LSP a letter of inquiry, to which LSP responded soothingly. OSHA accepted LSP's assurances without making any on-site investigation.

Early in March 1975, EPA routinely sent to LSP an inspector, whose concern was aroused. But the EPA's jurisdiction over dangerous pesticides hinged on whether the plant was producing a finished pesticide, as opposed to a mere pesticide component. Not sure whether he had jurisdiction to take any action, the inspector sent an inquiry to the EPA regional office in Philadelphia. From Philadelphia the inquiry was sent to the legal department and the registration department in Washington. The inquiry was unanswered and presumably was still kicking around Washington when the Commonwealth of Virginia closed the plant in July.

This series of events, or non-events, raises some of the most serious problems society faces. The share of services taken over by the public sector has increased geometrically in the past decades. Yet we have made no corresponding advance in figuring out how to increase the accountability of public agencies and their minions. How are we going to bring the law home to *them*? Prosecutions of public officials for their out-and-out criminal acts are rare enough. In the Kepone affair, not a single Hopewell official was ever indicted. And when it comes not to crimes but just to botching the jobs they are supposed to be doing, there is almost no type of real accountability whatsoever—perhaps a few uncomfortable moments before a Senate investigating committee after a dam has burst.

Can't We Do Better?

What can the law do to prevent such tragedies?

First, society and industry need a way to discover and analyze dangers of this sort well before they have reached the level of catastrophe. The new Toxic Substances Control Act, by requiring manufacturers to investigate and prepare extensive analyses on the risks of their products before marketing them, is one of the most positive steps in this direction.

But even under the best "early warning" system, not all such corporate-related tragedies are going to be averted. An early warning system tight enough to anticipate every technological threat would probably prove a social disaster. Thus we have to expect similar incidents in the future. How can we best handle the bureaucratic wrongdoers—not merely the business corporations, but the municipal corporations and public agencies also involved?

Let us begin with a statement of one of Allied's lawyers made in pleading for lenient treatment. The company, he told the court,

> has established a company-wide program to audit and analyze its environmental programs and the techniques that are being applied at all plants. And this is an on-going study and effort designed to

insure that not only the letter of the law is complied with, but the spirit of the law.

This sounds like exactly the effort we want every institutional law-breaker to undertake when it has felt the sting of the law. But what does it guarantee? What are the assurances that such an audit will be carried out and implemented thoroughly?

The key may be to apply the powers of probation more forcefully and imaginatively than heretofore. Judge Merhige might have been wise to require both Allied and Hopewell to file with the court's probation officer a report stating why, in view of each corporation's own "findings," the wrongful conduct was allowed to occur: What were the defects in internal policies, procedures, and organization?

Next, each corporation should have been required to propose its own recommendations as to the best way of assuring appropriate conduct in the future. Such measures might include:

1. Alterations in the organization's pattern of operation, including new standards for the monitoring of toxic-substance handling, medical examination of employees, etc.
2. Changes in personnel, including firings, suspensions, and hirings.
3. Establishment of new positions with specified tasks and responsibilities; in the case of Allied, liaisons with companies specially processing materials under contract.
4. Implementation of new information procedures designed to assure that appropriate data are adequately gathered and transmitted to corporate officers of appropriate authority.

Since the various public agencies involved were never convicted of any offense, they would not, strictly speaking, be subject to a court's probationary orders. But the court might still, in its discretion and invoking the weight of its authority, prod each of them to prepare papers of the same scope: Each agency would have to explain why it had not forestalled the tragedy and would set forth the measures it intended to prevent recurrence.

Then, the court might hold a hearing on the adequacy of each party's findings and proposals. If substantial controversy were anticipated, the court might also appoint a peer group review committee (as the SEC was appointed in the settlement of actions against accounting firms) to assess the organization's proposed control devices and help resolve disagreements.

Finally, when an acceptable and detailed probation order had been agreed to, each organization should be made to prepare and file with the court, every six or twelve months, a statement confirming its compliance with the obligations of the probation. The statement would be signed by designated supervisory personnel, who would be legally accountable if the representations were misleading.

Such a procedure—which is detailed in a model bill I have drafted that is presently being circulated among federal and state law-makers—is a less than perfect way to deal with the complex problems of an organizationally based society. But as a review of the Kepone affair suggests, it would be a major step in the right direction.

11 / Who's Burning Boston?

JAMES P. BRADY

. . . THIS CITY has experienced a "fire wave" of almost fantastic proportions in the last decade, with tremendous losses of life and property. These disasters have sometimes been the consequence of carelessness, decaying buildings, racial hatred, personal grudges, or vandalism; but it is increasingly apparent that many of them have been the result of what has become a major form of organized racketeering: arson for profit. Arson does not occur randomly in the city, but is closely associated with patterns of systematic speculation in transitional neighborhoods. The processs of "redlining," "block busting," and "gentrification" which accompany arson have destabilized many of the city's neighborhoods and intensified racial hostilities, while winning enormous profits for entrepreneurs, both criminal and "legitimate."

All evidence indicates that the experience of Boston, while perhaps extreme, is hardly unusual: Arson is fast becoming one of the most destructive and profitable crimes in the country. Its victims are not merely those driven from their homes, but whole communities; and its perpetrators are not only "torches," but also real estate companies, banks, and corrupt law enforcement, fire department, and insurance corporation personnel. The scale and complexity of this crime, which involves such respectable institutions and individuals alongside more recognizably "criminal" types, call into question the whole theoretical underpinning of deviance theory. . . .

The Spreading Arson Wave and the Failure of Control Measures

Arson is the end of a process of deterioration that has afflicted neighborhoods in most large cities for at least twenty years. The record shows that arson is the fastest-growing and one of the most destructive crimes in the country, easily ranking with the FBI's official index crimes. Over the period 1965–75 there was a 325 percent increase in known crimes of arson, and the law Enforcement Assistance Administration has reported that the rates are still rising. The

133

National Insurance Service Office confirms that an estimated $4 billion was paid directly by insurance companies for arson fires during 1976, while in 1979 there were over 148,500 known incidents of arson, with still higher losses. In Detroit over 10,000 homes were destroyed by arsonists in the decade. Arson rates in Los Angeles have risen 500 percent in the last five years, and they have climbed 300 percent in three years. These figures, it should be stressed, take into account only those fires positively classified by local fire departments as "incendiary" and do not include even larger losses to fires of "suspicious" or "undetermined" origins.

More than 1,000 people died in 1975 in arson fires, another 700 were burned to death in 1978, and another 675 died in 1979. Many of these were children or old people, unable to move quickly to escape the flames in the darkness. The buildings in which they died were typically unsafe, unhealthy, and in clear violation of fire and safety codes. "Death by fire" is a pauper's epitaph, as arsonists strike most often in inner-city districts of the poor. The "decline of the city" leads ultimately to zones like New York's South Bronx or Boston's Roxbury, where the scale of devastation can only be compared to the passing of earthquakes or blitzkreigs. We are witnessing the creation of a new geographic morphology: the urban desert.

One might think that insurance companies would press for stricter enforcement of arson laws, since the fires cost them millions of dollars in yearly claims. In fact, they simply pass these losses along to the consumer with higher premiums. The federal government's creation of "Fair Plan" coverage for inner-city districts also protects the companies, since they pay only a percentage of the losses. The companies, like the banks with which they are typically interlocked, sometimes finance the conversion of fire-ravaged blocks into condominiums or offices, with handsome profits. Arson has not been recognized as a major problem or given a high action priority by the insuring and lending institutions. . . .

The pattern of arson arrests, convictions, and investigations is dismal, and there have been a number of serious cases involving corrupt police in arson rings. While many thousands of set fires are wrongly recorded as "accidental," even those classified as arson receive little official notice. United States Fire Administration statistics reveal that fewer than 9 percent of all reported arsons lead to an arrest, with fewer than 1 percent cleared by conviction. Most of those persons caught and convicted are juveniles, pyromaniacs, or revenge-seeking individuals, rather than professional torches hired by property owners. Indeed, the dominant official view is that arson is a crime of passion, or an act of the feeble-minded or mentally unbalanced. This, of course, is consistent with racist and elitist views, since most arsons occur in poor and minority districts, where, presumably, "hot-headed," stupid, or perverted individuals are concentrated. . . .

Urban Speculation and the Arson Process

The decline of central city districts is often described as "decay" or "blight," but neither is really a fit image. Arson and slum conditions are not the conclusion of some organic process, but rather a political and economic one. The "urban deserts" are natural only in that they are the logical outcome of good business practice and the fruits of ruthless speculation. Fortunes are made through arson, particularly when burned buildings have been insured far beyond their real value or when they stand on land suddenly made more valuable by the coming of gentrification to the central city.

The connections between racketeering and legitimate businesses are hardly peculiar to arson. Virtually every student of white collar or organized crime has observed that corporate enterprises engage in economic crimes as a routine practice and that virtually all crime syndicates are linked to legitimate businesses. Sutherland was among the first to point out that price fixing, fraud, unfair labor practices, and tax evasion are routine in the business world, but that such offenses are in general not recognized or punished as criminal acts. The President's Crime Commission concluded that such crimes far exceed ordinary street crimes in frequency and damage. More recently, Grutzner, Reiman, Pearce, and Chambliss have demonstrated that the competitive dynamics of capitalism virtually demand that corporations engage in systematic violations of law in order to win government contracts, avoid taxes, control labor, and otherwise surpass their competitors in amassing profits. As Chambliss has shown so effectively in his studies of Seattle, the typical gangster syndicates are dominated by unseen participants from government and corporations, who provide capital and protection for the racketeers. The interests of these respectable elite members of the group are typically managed by underlings (who may even be uniformed police or lawyers), and the conscious involvement of members of the elite is minimal. So long as their investments prove sound and scandals are averted, they have little reason to question the successful policies of their subordinates.

As in other sorts of organized crime, the involvement of legitimate businesses in arson is indirect; bankers, especially, are most likely only dimly aware that bank policies both contribute to and profit from arson waves in the city. Unscrupulous landlords and real estate companies are more often consciously involved; indeed, some specialize in acquiring "fire prone" buildings, which they promptly insure at artificially high levels. Of course the professional torch who sets the fire, and the corrupt insurance adjuster, fire code inspector, and police detectives who may conceal the fraud are well aware of their crimes. Yet, as in other rackets, it is the unseen, indirect (even unaware) participants who make millions from arson, while the various underlings count their share in hundreds of dollars. In the unlikely event of serious investigation it is consistently the subordinate criminals who will go to prison. Bankers and realtors, whose legal resources are better and who face charges less serious, may be publicly embarrassed, but rarely are they given criminal sentences. The recent Symphony Road arson conspiracy in Boston is a case in point. The banks unwittingly created the motive for arson, through investment and credit practices deflating property values and prompting worried landlords to plan a fire as an escape from a bad investment. The banks profit in the same way when arson-prone buyers take unwanted foreclosed properties off their hands and handsomely repay the second mortgage with part of the fire claim settlement from the overinsured building. Banks and realtors also profit from fires which clear tenants and gut interiors to ease the lucrative conversion of tenements into condominiums. Again, individual landlords and corrupt officials make large profits, but the banks and realtors may gain the most from the financing and resale of property, without fully realizing their own contribution to the arson process. We must consider here two main paths to arson, which depend upon whether the target neighborhood is headed for economic decline or resurgence. In both instances the profits to be made from fires can be staggering. I will outline each of the two processes in brief, starting with that in the declining neighborhood.

Banks, seeking to maximize profits from investment, shift their capital to favor loans in high-yield areas while avoiding poorer districts which they regard as risky. In the unfavored or "redlined" areas, they act, informally, to discourage mortgage applications and to deny credit for home improvement or business loans. Consequently, it becomes more difficult to maintain or sell a home or small business, and property values fall. Redlining continues despite the passage of neighborhood reinvestment laws, both because the banks are more secretive in their practices and because bank mergers grant banking chains greater legal discretion for allotting funds within their enlarged depositor home districts. Property owners, unable to sell or maintain their buildings without available credit and worried about falling values, increasingly turn to arson in order to recover their investment.

While redlining banks only contribute indirectly to arson by worried landlords, some banks themselves profit through their sale of foreclosed properties to known and repeated arsonists. The resale of foreclosed properties in unattractive (often redlined) districts is a major problem for lending institutions. Falling real estate values often make it difficult to find a new purchaser for deteriorated buildings. A backlog of property taxes, which must be paid to gain a clear property title, is an additional and often expensive complication. Thus, legitimate buyers may offer only a fraction of the money lost by the bank in the first mortgage, and soaring rehabilitation costs and new taxes make investment prospects dimmer still.

Enter the arson-prone investor, who purchases the property at well above its real value. The law specifies that, in the event of total loss by fire, the holder of the initial mortgage (the bank) is first paid from any insurance settlement. Thus the bank makes good its initial bad investment, and the owners profit from the difference between the mortgage and the buildings' (higher) appraised and insured value. This arrangement may be aided by bribery of bank appraisers or insurance adjusters. Quick repayment from insurance claims is typical in many states specifying a thirty- or forty-five-day limit, unless the insurer can show probable cause for criminal investigation. Given the record of arson enforcement, there is every prospect of substantial earnings by the arsonist and easy recovery by the bank. The end of the process is the same, whether this is a result of negligence by the bank or outright corruption.

A recently investigated Boston institution, the South Boston Savings Bank, illustrates this point. During the period 1970–77 the bank foreclosed on a total of seventy-six parcels, many of them in depressed neighborhoods. Over this period thirty-nine of these foreclosed properties suffered a total of seventy-nine fires, averaging about two fires per parcel in the last seven years. These may be compared with sixty-nine properties foreclosed by the Veteran's Administration and Housing and Urban Development, in which new mortgages were issued in the same high-risk neighborhoods and to owners who (unlike the bank's debtors) were required to make only minimal down payments; in this group there were thirty-six fires at twenty-six addresses. The timing of the fires in the Boston bank's property makes the incidents appear more suspicious. One would expect more fires to occur in the year before foreclosure, when owners might turn to desperate means, and fewer fires once foreclosure passes and new owners try to rehabilitate the property. This is precisely the pattern observed in the houses foreclosed by the Veteran's Administration and Housing and Urban Development. However, the bank's new owners seemed to have especially "bad luck," with the greatest number of fires occurring in the first year after resale.

Ten of the torched properties were sold to Oster Development Corporation, one of whose officers had been arrested and confined for arson-linked murders in Newton; and five were sold to George Lincoln, recently convicted of over a dozen arson crimes in the Symphony Road district. Four others indicted on the basis of Lincoln's testimony also held mortgages on property previously foreclosed by the same bank. Russel Tardanico, whose properties burned twenty-one times in the period 1972–77 (with tremendous losses), had been convicted of arson in 1970. Several firemen were injured in one of the most recent incendiary fires. Tardanico explained, "If you own a lot of property, you have a lot of fires, you have a lot of broken windows and leaky roofs."

Real estate companies also exploit the shaken confidence of residents in redlined districts in order to encourage panic selling at prices well below real values. Racism is often consciously manipulated as brokers circulate rumors of large-scale movement to the neighborhoods by blacks, with dramatic crime increases and catastrophic declines in property values. Once the flight of white residents begins, the process of quick sale and resale yields tremendous profits, especially since many of the first buyers are hired by the real estate companies themselves. In order to accelerate turnover, realtors may encourage new owners to seek Federal Housing Administration loans which require only minimal down payments and offer attractive housing rehabilitation credits. A recent United States Senate investigation of the Boston-area Federal Housing Administration program found "widespread collusion between unscrupulous brokers and corrupt FHA appraisers." This process of "blockbusting" yields enormous profits at the risk of very light and infrequently imposed penalties.

The identification of those ultimately responsible for arson is made more difficult by beneficiaries' widespread practice of listing "straws," or dummy owners or holding companies, to conceal the names of those who will ultimately profit from fires. A recent investigation of one such straw in the declining Dorchester district of Boston is illustrative. . . . The straw in this example, named "Sarah Cutler," was also known as "Leona Kantrowicz" or "Kantrowicz and Kantrowicz." Properties owned by this person are remarkable for their huge unpaid tax bills and their uncanny tendency to burn in fires described by fire department investigators as "incendiary" or "suspicious." Interestingly, income from insurance premiums did not go to "Cutler/Kantrowicz" but rather to the "Sarah Cutler" Trust. The beneficiaries of that trust were Albert Kline and John Kerrigan. The former is the insurance broker of recently convicted landlord/arsonist Michael Lombroso, while the latter is a former member of the Boston School Committee and a leading politician.

. . . The damage caused by arson can range from total destruction of property to relatively minor losses. The biggest, most dramatic fires can be the final solution for unscrupulous landlords as well as banks holding foreclosed properties. Smaller fires can also be a source of profit if owners pocket claims settlements and then arrange for incomplete or fraudulent repairs to be covered through another larger fire. Bribery of housing inspectors and insurance adjusters is often a part of this tactic. This was precisely the method used by convicted arsonists Lincoln and Tardanico, who were also their own repair contractors.

Although arson is most commonly associated with declining neighborhoods, as in the above examples, increasingly evident is a pattern of "fire for profit" associated with sharply rising property values in resurgent urban districts. The movement of professionals and prosperous small businesses from the suburbs back into central cities has meant sharply increased land values in the process known as gentrification. The problem, from the speculators' point of view, is that many of the buildings are already occupied by low-income tenants, who may be protected by leases or even by statutory limits on rent increases or evictions without cause.

In Boston, the process of gentrification has led to soaring property values, and the conversion by landlords of tenements into condominiums has yielded unprecedented profits. However, old tenants may be evicted for conversion purposes only after a two-year waiting period, and substantial rent increases may be contested in public hearings. If tenants leave, their vacant apartments are "decontrolled"; but few willingly put themselves at the mercy of a housing market characterized by low availability and high rents. In this situation, the prospects of quick and enormous profits often tempt impatient landlords without legitimate grievances to push out old tenants through other means.

Once again fire is a common solution. As the arson investigator for First Security Corporation noted, "There are three basic upfront advantages that even a relatively unsophisticated building owner might recognize in having a friendly fire on the premises: rendering the property uninhabitable, facilitating renovation by gutting the interior, and generating insurance money to finance reconversion." The record of recent arsons in Boston's prime "conversion districts" certainly bears this out. In 1980 arson rates increased by 400 percent in the Back Bay area, where property values are sky rocketing and bank mortgages are easily obtained. Investigators from the federally funded Urban Educational Systems show that the pattern of arson closely reflects conversion plans for the district. The district fire chief voiced a suspicion that a similar pattern of arsons corresponded with condominium conversions in the Brighton area. City Councilman Ray

Flynn, after reading the evidence in recent municipal housing hearings, concluded,

> I am convinced that there is a correlation between building conversions and arson. There is nothing so effective as fire for circumventing eviction procedures. Just look at the money being made by conversions. It is second only to the lottery in the amount you can make in one shot.

A number of recent court cases have pitted tenants against owners of arson-prone buildings in prime conversion districts. Robert Ward of Brookline was recently convicted of setting fire to tenants' apartments in one of his Back Bay buildings; and the district attorney cited condominium conversion profits as the central motive. In civil actions elsewhere, tenants of the well-known Beacon Chambers rooming house and numerous apartment houses in Beacon Hill, Back Bay, and Brighton won injunctions against eviction in buildings landlords had declared "condemned" following suspicious fires and systematic negligence. The ironic courtroom debate is between landlords who insist that their buildings have been rendered uninhabitable and tenants who disagree and want to continue paying rent. These patterns within resurgent districts are a new sort of arson, and appear likely to increase as the conflict between landlords' and tenants' interests intensifies and regulatory statutes hamper unrestricted profit making.

Arson, then, is a complex crime, bringing direct and indirect earnings to both legitimate enterprises and criminal entrepreneurs. Taxpayers must pay for fraudulent claims through the federally subsidized Fair Plan and legitimate property owners and small businesses in the arson-ravaged district also suffer losses. Tenants in the torched buildings, whose possessions are usually uninsured, forfeit their property and often their lives. . . .

Additional Readings

Block, Alan A. and Frank R. Scarpitti. *Poisoning for Profit: The Mafia and Toxic Waste in America*. New York: Morrow, 1985.

Brady, James. "Arson, Urban Economy, and Organized Crime: The Case of Boston." *Social Problems* 31 (October 1983): 1–27.

Brown, Michael H. *Laying Waste: The Poisoning of America by Toxic Chemicals*. New York: Pantheon, 1980.

Diperna, Paula. *Cluster Mystery: Epidemic and the Children of Woburn, Mass.* St. Louis: Mosby, 1985.

Epstein, Samuel S., Lester O. Brown, and Carl Pope. *Hazardous Waste in America*. San Francisco: Sierra Club Books, 1982.

Erikson, Kai. *Everything in Its Path: Destruction of Community in the Buffalo Creek Flood*. New York: Simon and Schuster, 1976.

Etzkowitz, Henry. "Corporate Induced Disaster: Three Mile Island and the Delegitimation of Nuclear Power." *Humanity and Society* 8 (August 1984): 228–52.

Ford, Daniel F. *Three Mile Island: Thirty Minutes to Meltdown*. New York: Penguin Books, 1982.

Levine, Adeline. *Love Canal: Science, Politics, and People*. Lexington, Mass.: Lexington Books, 1982.

Tolchin, Susan J. and Martin Tolchin. "Political Meltdown: Reactors, Risks and Regulation." In *The Big Business Reader: On Corporate America*, edited by Mark Green. New York: Pilgrim Press, 1983.

Sethi, S. Prakash. "The Santa Barbara Oil Spill." In *Corporate and Governmental Deviance*, 2d ed., edited by M. David Ermann and Richard J. Lundman. New York: Oxford University Press, 1982.

Part IV

Voices from the Corporate Bureaucracy

KERMIT VANDIVIER worked as an engineering lab analyst for the B.F. Goodrich Company reviewing test data on aircraft brakes the company was designing for the new A7D light attack airplane. In the article "Why Should My Conscience Bother Me?," Vandivier relates the cover-up of fraudulent lab data by Goodrich officials to conceal dangerous safety defects in the brake design, and the self-serving rationalizations by company executives to neutralize any feelings of guilt for their actions. Admitting his own initial complicity in the cover-up, Vandivier, who subsequently became a whistle-blower and government witness against Goodrich, describes the immense managerial pressure on everyone involved to go along with the deception, even at the risk of jeopardizing the lives of test pilots who might fly the planes with the malfunctioning brakes.

In the article "Benton Harlow: Distributor of Unsafe Drugs," sociologist James Carey presents excerpts from his interview with a former executive of a large American pharmaceutical company. Harlow was part of a conspiracy of company executives who were convicted of fraud and lying to the Food and Drug Administration about the results of animal laboratory studies testing the effects of an anticholesterol drug the company was developing. Among the frightening side effects of this drug were eye cataracts, hair loss, and painful dryness of the skin. Carey provides an insightful analysis of the manner in which Harlow and his colleagues drifted into this cover-up and the apparent lack of any opposition or even moral qualms at the prospect of marketing the unsafe drug. Such law violations were instead rationalized as "part and parcel of the hazards inherent in discovering and marketing new drugs." As Carey points out, many company executives like Benton Harlow are apt to view their behavior not as criminal but as "technically illegal"—risky but

143

often necessary for the survival of the company under conditions of "cutthroat competition."

It takes uncommon courage to be a whistle-blower and to risk one's career for exposing corporate wrongdoing. As the two senior engineers who testified before the presidential commission investigating the space shuttle Challenger disaster discovered, corporate executives who go public are often punished—not rewarded—for acting on their ethical principles to challenge management decisions that may compromise human safety for lucrative government contracts. This is also true in the nuclear energy industry, where Peter Faulkner recounts his experiences in the final article of this section, "Exposing Risks of Nuclear Disaster."

Faulkner, a systems engineer for the Nuclear Services Corporation, describes his frustrating encounters with both his own company and government regulatory agencies when he exposed engineering deficiencies and defects in nuclear power systems already on the market. Fired from his job and blackballed by the entire nuclear industry, Faulkner bravely attempted to warn citizens about nuclear industry problems, but found that the government and industry were more interested in promoting nuclear technology than in protecting public safety. In the shadow of the disasters at Three Mile Island and Chernobyl, Faulkner raises some penetrating questions regarding not only the present safety of nuclear technology, but also the gradual abdication of any moral responsibility by industry engineers who, partly out of fear for their jobs, "obediently and unquestioningly" refuse to challenge managerial decisions that often place more value on profits or bureaucratic goals than on human lives.

12 / Why Should My Conscience Bother Me?

KERMIT VANDIVIER

The B. F. Goodrich Co. is what business magazines like to speak of as "a major American corporation." It has operations in a dozen states and as many foreign countries, and of these far-flung facilities, the Goodrich plant at Troy, Ohio, is not the most imposing. It is a small, one-story building, once used to manufacture airplanes. Set in the grassy flatlands of west-central Ohio, it employs only about six hundred people. Nevertheless, it is one of the three largest manufacturers of aircraft wheels and brakes, a leader in a most profitable industry. Goodrich wheels and brakes support such well-known planes as the F111, the C5A, the Boeing 727, the XB70 and many others. Its customers include almost every aircraft manufacturer in the world.

Contracts for aircraft wheels and brakes often run into millions of dollars, and ordinarily a contract with a total value of less than $70,000, though welcome, would not create any special stir of joy in the hearts of Goodrich sales personnel. But purchase order P-23718, issued on June 18, 1967, by the LTV Aerospace Corporation, and ordering 202 brake assemblies for a new Air Force plane at a total price of $69,417, was received by Goodrich with considerable glee. And there was good reason. Some ten years previously, Goodrich had built a brake for LTV that was, to say the least, considerably less than a rousing success. The brake had not lived up to Goodrich's promises, and after experiencing considerable difficulty, LTV had written off Goodrich as a source of brakes. Since that time, Goodrich salesmen had been unable to sell so much as a shot of brake fluid to LTV. So in 1967, when LTV requested bids on wheels and brakes for the new A7D light attack aircraft it proposed to build for the Air Force,

Goodrich submitted a bit that was absurdly low, so low that LTV could not, in all prudence, turn it down.

Goodrich had, in industry parlance, "bought into the business." Not only did the company not expect to make a profit on the deal; it was prepared, if necessary, to lose money. For aircraft brakes are not something that can be ordered off the shelf. They are designed for a particular aircraft, and once an aircraft manufacturer buys a brake, he is forced to purchase all replacement parts from the brake manufacturer. The $70,000 that Goodrich would get for making the brake would be a drop in the bucket when compared with the cost of the linings and other parts the Air Force would have to buy from Goodrich during the lifetime of the aircraft. Furthermore, the company which manufactures brakes for one particular model of an aircraft quite naturally has the inside track to supply other brakes when the planes are updated and improved.

Thus, that first contract, regardless of the money involved, is very important, and Goodrich, when it learned that it had been awarded the A7D contract, was determined that while it may have slammed the door on its own foot ten years before, this time, the second time around, things would be different. The word was soon circulated throughout the plant: "We can't bungle it this time. We've got to give them a good brake, regardless of the cost."

There was another factor which had undoubtedly influenced LTV. All aircraft brakes made today are of the disk type, and the bid submitted by Goodrich called for a relatively small brake, one containing four disks and weighing only 106 pounds. The weight of any aircraft part is extremely important. The lighter a part is, the heavier the plane's payload can be. The four-rotor, 106-pound brake promised by Goodrich was about as light as could be expected, and this undoubtedly had helped move LTV to award the contract to Goodrich.

The brake was designed by one of Goodrich's most capable engineers, John Warren. A tall, lanky blond and a graduate of Purdue, Warren had come from the Chrysler Corporation seven years before and had become adept at aircraft brake design. The happy-go-lucky manner he usually maintained belied a temper which exploded whenever anyone ventured to offer any criticism of his work, no matter how small. On these occasions, Warren would turn red in the face, often throwing or slamming something and then stalking from the scene. As his co-workers learned the consequences of criticizing him, they did so less and less readily, and when he submitted his preliminary design for the A7D brake, it was accepted without question.

Warren was named project engineer for the A7D, and he, in turn, assigned the task of producing the final production design to a newcomer to the Goodrich engineering stable, Searle Lawson. Just turned twenty-six, Lawson had been out of the Northrup Institute of Technology only one year when he came to Goodrich in January 1967. Like Warren, he had worked for a while in the automotive industry, but his engineering degree was in aeronautical and astronautical sciences, and when the opportunity came to enter his special field, via Goodrich, he took it. At the Troy plant, Lawson had been assigned to various "paper projects" to break him in, and after several months spent reviewing statistics and old brake designs, he was beginning to fret at the lack of challenge. When told he was being assigned to his first "real" project, he was elated and immediately plunged into his work.

The major portion of the design had already been completed by Warren, and major assemblies for the brake had already been ordered from Goodrich suppliers. Naturally, however, before Goodrich could start making the brakes on a production basis, much testing would have to be done. Lawson would have to determine the best materials to use for the linings and discover what minor adjustments in the design would have to be made.

Then, after the preliminary testing and after the brake was judged ready for production, one whole brake assembly would undergo a series of grueling, simulated braking stops and other severe trials called qualification tests. These tests are required by the military, which gives very detailed specifications on how they are to be conducted, the criteria for failure, and so on. They are performed in the Goodrich plant's test laboratory, where huge machines called dynamometers can simulate the weight and speed of almost any aircraft. After the brakes pass the laboratory tests, they are approved for production, but before the brakes are accepted for use in military service, they must undergo further extensive flight tests.

Searle Lawson was well aware that much work had to be done before the A7D brake could go into production, and he knew that LTV had set the last two weeks in June, 1968, as the starting dates for flight tests. So he decided to begin testing immediately. Goodrich's suppliers had not yet delivered the brake housing and other parts, but the brake disks had arrived, and using the housing from a brake similar in size and weight to the A7D brake, Lawson built a prototype. The prototype was installed in a test wheel and placed on one of the big dynamometers in the plant's test laboratory. The dynamometer was adjusted to simulate the weight of the A7D and Lawson began a series of tests "landing" the wheel and brake at the A7D's landing speed, and braking it to a stop. The main purpose of these preliminary tests was to learn what temperatures would develop within the brake during the simulated stops and to evaluate the lining materials tentatively selected for use.

During a normal aircraft landing the temperatures inside the brake may reach 1000 degrees, and occasionally a bit higher. During Lawson's first simulated landings, the temperature of his prototype brake reached 1500 degrees. The brake glowed a bright cherry-red and threw off incandescent particles of metal and lining material as the temperature reached its peak. After a few such stops, the brake was dismantled and the linings were found to be almost completely disintegrated. Lawson called this first failure up to chance and, ordering new lining materials, tried again.

The second attempt was a repeat of the first. The brake became extremely hot, causing the lining materials to crumble into dust.

After the third such failure, Lawson, inexperienced though he was, knew that the fault lay not in defective parts or unsuitable lining material but in the basic design of the brake itself. Ignoring Warren's original computations, Lawson made his own, and it didn't take him long to discover where the trouble lay—the brake was too small. There simply was not enough surface area on the disk to stop the aircraft without generating the excessive heat that caused the linings to fail.

The answer to the problem was obvious but far from simple—the four-disk brake would have to be scrapped, and a new design, using five disks, would have to be developed. The implications were not lost on Lawson. Such a step would require the junking of all the four-disk-brake subassemblies, many of which had now begun to arrive from the various suppliers. It would also mean several weeks of preliminary design and testing and many more weeks of waiting while the suppliers made and delivered the new subassemblies.

Yet, several weeks had already gone by since LTV's order had arrived, and the date for delivery of the first production brakes for flight testing was only a few months away.

Although project engineer John Warren had more or less turned the A7D over to Lawson, he knew of the difficulties Lawson had been experiencing. He had assured the young engineer that the problem revolved around getting the right kind of lining material. Once that was found, he said, the difficulties would end.

Despite the evidence of the abortive tests and Lawson's careful computations, Warren rejected the suggestion that the four-disk brake was too light for the job. Warren knew that his superior had already told LTV, in rather glowing terms, that the preliminary tests on the A7D brake were very successful. Indeed, Warren's superiors weren't aware at this time of the troubles on the brake. It would have been difficult for Warren to admit not only that he had made a serious error in his calculations and original design but that his mistakes had been caught by a green kid, barely out of college.

Warren's reaction to a five-disk brake was not unexpected by Lawson, and, seeing that the four-disk brake was not to be abandoned so easily, he took his calculations and dismal test results one step up the corporate ladder.

At Goodrich, the man who supervises the engineers working on projects slated for production is called, predictably, the projects manager. The job was held by a short, chubby and bald man named Robert Sink. A man truly devoted to his work, Sink was as likely to be found at his desk at ten o'clock on Sunday night as ten o'clock on Monday morning. His outside interests consisted mainly of tinkering on a Model-A Ford and an occasional game of golf. Some fifteen years before, Sink had begun working at Goodrich as a lowly draftsman. Slowly, he worked his way up. Despite his geniality, Sink was neither respected nor liked by the majority of the engineers, and his appointment as their supervisor did not improve their feelings about him. They thought he had only gone to high school. It quite naturally rankled those who had gone through years of college and acquired impressive specialties such as thermodynamics and astronautics to be commanded by a man whom they considered their intellectual inferior. But, though Sink had no college training, he had something even more useful: a fine working knowledge of company politics.

Puffing upon a Meerschaum pipe, Sink listened gravely as young Lawson confided his fears about the four-disk brake. Then he examined Lawson's calculations and the results of the abortive tests. Despite the fact that he was not a qualified engineer, in the strictest sense of the word, it must certainly have been obvious to Sink that Lawson's calculations were correct and that a four-disk brake would never have worked on the A7D.

But other things of equal importance were also obvious. First, to concede that Lawson's calculations were correct would also mean conceding that Warren's calculations were incorrect. As projects manager, he not only was responsible for Warren's activities, but, in admitting that Warren had erred, he would have to admit that he had erred in trusting Warren's judgment. It also meant that, as projects manager, it would be he who would have to explain the whole messy situation to the Goodrich hierarchy, not only at Troy but possibly on the corporate level at Goodrich's Akron offices. And, having taken Warren's judgment of the four-disk brake at face value (he was forced to do this since, not being an engineer, he was unable to exercise any engineering judgment of his own), he had assured LTV, not once but several times, that about all there was left to do on the brake was pack it in a crate and ship it out the back door.

There's really no problem at all, he told Lawson. After all, Warren was an experienced engineer, and if he said the brake would work, it would work. Just keep on testing and probably, maybe even on the very next try, it'll work out just fine.

Lawson was far from convinced, but without the support of his superiors there was little he could do except keep on testing. By now, housings for the four-disk brake had begun to arrive at the plant, and Lawson was able to build up a production model of the brake and begin the formal qualification tests demanded by the military.

The first qualification attempts went exactly as the tests on the prototype had. Terrific heat developed within the brakes and, after a few, short, simulated stops, the linings crumbled. A new type of lining material was ordered and once again an attempt to qualify the brake was made. Again, failure.

Experts were called in from lining manufacturers, and new lining "mixes" were tried, always with the same result. Failure.

It was now the last week in March 1968, and flight tests were scheduled to begin in seventy days. Twelve separate attempts had been made to formally qualify the brake, and all had failed. It was no longer possible for anyone to ignore the glaring truth that the brake was a dismal failure and that nothing short of a major design change could ever make it work.

In the engineering department, panic set in. A glum-faced Lawson prowled the test laboratory dejectedly. Occasionally, Warren would witness some simulated stop on the brake and, after it was completed, troop silently back to his desk. Sink, too, showed an unusual interest in the trials, and he and Warren would converse in low tones while poring over the results of the latest tests. Even the most inexperienced of the lab technicians and the men who operated the testing equipment knew they had a "bad" brake on their hands, and there was some grumbling about "wasting time on a brake that won't work."

New menaces appeared. An engineering team from LTV arrived at the plant to get a good look at the brake in action. Luckily, they stayed only a few days, and Goodrich engineers managed to cover the true situation without too much difficulty.

On April 4, the thirteenth attempt at qualification was begun. This time no attempt was made to conduct the tests by the methods and techniques spelled out in the military specifications. Regardless of how it had to be done, the brake was to be "nursed" through the required fifty simulated stops.

Fans were set up to provide special cooling. Instead of maintaining pressure on the brake until the test wheel had come to a complete stop, the pressure was reduced when the wheel had decelerated to around 15 mph, allowing it to "coast" to a stop. After each stop, the brake was diassembled and carefully cleaned, and after some of the stops, internal brake parts were machined in order to remove warp and other disfigurations caused by the high heat.

By these and other methods, all clearly contrary to the techniques established by the military specifications, the brake was coaxed through the fifty stops. But even using these methods, the brake could not meet all the requirements. On one stop the wheel rolled for a distance of 16,000 feet, nearly three miles, before the brake could bring it to a stop. The normal distance required for such a stop was around 3500 feet.

On April 11, the day the thirteenth test was completed, I became personally involved in the A7D situation.

I had worked in the Goodrich test laboratory for five years, starting first as an instrumentation engineer, then later becoming a data analyst and technical writer. As part of my duties, I analyzed the reams and reams of instrumentation data that came from the many testing machines in the laboratory, then transcribed it to a more usable form for the engineering department. And when a new-type brake had successfully completed the required qualification tests, I would issue a formal qualification report.

Qualification reports were an accumulation of all the data and test logs compiled by the test technicians during the qualification tests, and were documentary proof that a brake had met all the requirements established by the military specifications and was therefore presumed safe for flight testing. Before actual flight tests were conducted on a brake, qualification reports had to be delivered to the customer and to various government officials.

On April 11, I was looking over the data from the latest A7D test, and I noticed that many irregularities in testing methods had been noted on the test logs.

Technically, of course, there was nothing wrong with conducting tests in any manner desired, so long as the test was for research purposes only. But qualification test methods are clearly delineated by the military, and I knew that this test had been a formal qualification attempt. One particular notation on the test logs caught my eye. For some of the stops, the instrument which recorded the brake pressure had been deliberately miscalibrated so that, while the brake pressure used during the stops was recorded as 1000 psi (the maximum pressure that would be available on the A7D aircraft), the pressure had actually been 1100 psi.

I showed the test logs to the test lab supervisor, Ralph Gretzinger, who said he had learned from the technician who had miscalibrated the instrument that he had been asked to do so by Lawson. Lawson, said Gretzinger, readily admitted asking for the miscalibration, saying he had been told to do so by Sink.

I asked Gretzinger why anyone would want to miscalibrate the data-recording instruments.

"Why? I'll tell you why," he snorted. "That brake is a failure. It's way too small for the job, and they're not ever going to get it to work. They're getting desperate, and instead of scrapping the damned thing and starting over, they figure they can horse around down here in the lab and qualify it that way."

An expert engineer, Gretzinger had been responsible for several innovations in brake design. It was he who had invented the unique brake system used on the famous XB70. A graduate of Georgia Tech, he was a stickler for detail and he had some very firm ideas about honesty and ethics. "If you want to find out what's going on," said Gretzinger, "ask Lawson, he'll tell you."

Curious, I did ask Lawson the next time he came into the lab. He seemed eager to discuss the A7D and gave me the history of his months of frustrating efforts to get Warren and Sink to change the brake design. "I just can't believe this is really happening," said Lawson, shaking his head slowly. "This isn't engineering, at least not what I thought it would be. Back in school, I thought that when you were an engineer, you tried to do your best, no matter what it cost. But this is something else."

He sat across the desk from me, his chin propped in his hand. "Just wait," he warned. "You'll get a chance to see what I'm talking about. You're going to get in the act too, because I've already had the word that we're going to make one more attempt to qualify the brake, and that's it. Win or lose, we're going to issue a qualification report!"

I reminded him that a qualification report could only be issued after a brake had successfully met all military requirements, and therefore, unless the next qualification attempt was a success, no report would be issued.

"You'll find out," retorted Lawson. "I was already told that regardless of what the brake does on test, it's going to be qualified." He said he had been told in those exact words at a conference with Sink and Russell Van Horn.

This was the first indication that Sink had brought his boss, Van Horn, into the mess. Although Van Horn, as manager of the design engineering section, was responsible for the entire department, he was not necessarily familiar with all phases of every project, and it was not uncommon for those under him to exercise the what-he-doesn't-know-won't-hurt-him philosophy. If he was aware of the full extent of the A7D situation, it meant that matters had truly reached a desperate stage—that Sink had decided not only to call for help but was looking toward that moment when blame must be borne and, if possible, shared.

Also, if Van Horn had said, "regardless what the brake does on test, it's going to be qualified," then it could only mean that, if necessary, a false qualification report would be issued! I discussed this possibility with Gretzinger, and he assured me that under no circumstances would such a report ever be issued.

"If they want a qualification report, we'll write them one, but we'll tell it just like it is," he declared emphatically. "No false data or false reports are going to come out of this lab."

On May 2, 1968, the fourteenth and final attempt to qualify the brake was begun. Although the same improper methods used to nurse the brake through the previous tests were employed, it soon became obvious that this too would end in failure.

When the tests were about half completed, Lawson asked if I would start preparing the various engineering curves and graphic displays which were normally incorporated in a qualification report. "It looks as though you'll be writing a qualification report shortly," he said.

I flatly refused to have anything to do with the matter and immediately told Gretzinger what I had been asked to do. He was furious and repeated his previous declaration that under no circumstances would any false data or other matter be issued from the lab.

"I'm going to get this settled right now, once and for all," he declared. "I'm going to see Line [Russell Line, manager of the Goodrich Technical Services Section, of which the test lab was a part] and find out just how far this thing is going to go!" He stormed out of the room.

In about an hour, he returned and called me to his desk. He sat silently for a few moments, then muttered, half to himself, "I wonder what the hell they'd do if I just quit?" I didn't answer and I didn't ask him what he meant. I knew. He had been beaten down. He had reached the point when the decision had to be made. Defy them now while there was still time—or knuckle under, sell out.

"You know," he went on uncertainly, looking down at his desk, "I've been an engineer for a long time, and I've always believed that ethics and integrity were every bit as important as theorems and formulas, and never once has anything happened to change my beliefs. Now this. . . . Hell, I've got two sons I've got to put through school and I just . . ." His voice trailed off.

He sat for a few more minutes, then, looking over the top of his glasses, said hoarsely, "Well, it looks like we're licked. The way it stands now, we're to go ahead and prepare the data and other things for the graphic presentation in the report, and when we're finished, someone upstairs will actually write the report."

"After all," he continued, "we're just drawing some curves, and what happens to them after they leave here, well, we're not responsible for that."

He was trying to persuade himself that as long as we were concerned with only one part of the puzzle and didn't see the completed picture, we really weren't doing anything wrong. He didn't believe what he was saying, and he knew I didn't believe it either. It was an embarrassing and shameful moment for both of us.

I wasn't at all satisfied with the situation and decided that I too would discuss the matter with Russell Line, the senior executive in our section.

Tall, powerfully built, his teeth flashing white, his face tanned to a coffee-brown by a daily stint with a sun lamp, Line looked and acted every inch the executive. He was a crossword-puzzle enthusiast and an ardent golfer, and though he had lived in Troy only a short time, he had been accepted into the Troy Country Club and made an official of the golf committee. He had been transferred from the Akron offices some two years previously, and an air of mystery surrounded him. Some office gossips figured he had been sent to Troy as the result of some sort of demotion. Others speculated that since the present general manager of the Troy plant was due shortly for retirement, Line had been transferred to Troy to assume that job and was merely occupying his present position to "get the feel of things." Whatever the case, he commanded great respect and had come to be well liked by those of us who worked under him.

He listened sympathetically while I explained how I felt about the A7D situation, and when I had finished, he asked me what I wanted him to do about it. I said that as employees of the Goodrich Company we had a responsibility to protect the company and its reputation if at all possible. I said I was certain that officers on the corporate level would never knowingly allow such tactics as had been employed on the A7D.

"I agree with you," he remarked, "but I still want to know what you want me to do about it."

I suggested that in all probability the chief engineer at the Troy plant, H. C. "Bud" Sunderman, was unaware of the A7D problem and that he, Line, should tell him what was going on.

Line laughed, good-humoredly. "Sure, I could, but I'm not going to. Bud probably already knows about this thing anyway, and if he doesn't, I'm sure not going to be the one to tell him."

"But why?"

"Because it's none of my business, and it's none of yours. I learned a long time ago not to worry about things over which I had no control. I have no control over this."

I wasn't satisfied with this answer, and I asked him if his conscience wouldn't bother him if, say, during flight tests on the brake, something should happen resulting in death or injury to the test pilot.

"Look," he said, becoming somewhat exasperated, "I just told you I have no control over this thing. Why should my conscience bother me?"

His voice took on a quiet, soothing tone as he continued. "You're just getting all upset over this thing for nothing. I just do as I'm told, and I'd advise you to do the same."

He had made his decision, and now I had to make mine.

I made no attempt to rationalize what I had been asked to do. It made no difference who would falsify which part of the report or whether the actual falsification would be by misleading numbers or misleading words. Whether by acts of commission or omission, all of us who contributed to the fraud would be guilty. The only question left for me to decide was whether or not I would become a party to the fraud.

Before coming to Goodrich in 1963, I had held a variety of jobs, each a little more pleasant, a little more rewarding than the last. At forty-two, with seven children, I had decided that the Goodrich Company would probably be my "home" for the rest of my working life. The job paid well, it was pleasant and challenging, and the future looked reasonably bright. My wife and I had bought a home and we were ready to settle down into a comfortable, middle-age, middle-class rut. If I refused to take part in the A7D fraud, I would have to either resign or be fired. The report would be written by someone anyway, but I would have the satisfaction of knowing I had had no part in the matter. But bills aren't paid with personal satisfaction, nor house payments with ethical principles. I made my decision. The next morning, I telephoned Lawson and told him I was ready to begin on the qualification report.

In a few minutes, he was at my desk, ready to begin. Before we started, I asked him, "Do you realize what we are going to do?"

"Yeah," he replied bitterly, "we're going to screw LTV. And speaking of screwing," he continued, "I know now how a whore feels, because that's exactly what I've become, an engineering whore. I've sold myself. It's all I can do to look at myself in the mirror when I shave. I make me sick."

I was surprised at his vehemence. It was obvious that he too had done his share of soul-searching and didn't like what he had found. Somehow, though, the air seemed clearer after his outburst, and we began working on the report.

I had written dozens of qualification reports, and I knew what a "good" one looked like. Resorting to the actual test data only on occasion, Lawson and I proceeded to prepare page after page of elaborate, detailed engineering curves, charts, and test logs, which purported to show what had happened during the formal qualification tests. Where temperatures were too high, we deliberately chopped them down a few hundred degrees, and where they were too low, we raised them to a value that would appear reasonable to the LTV and military engineers. Brake pressure, torque values, distances, times—everything of consequence was tailored to fit the occasion.

Occasionally, we would find that some test either hadn't been performed at all or had been conducted improperly. On those occasions, we "conducted" the test—successfully, of course—on paper.

For nearly a month we worked on the graphic presentation that would be part of the report. Meanwhile, the fourteenth and final qualification attempt had been completed, and the brake, not unexpectedly, had failed again.

During that month, Lawson and I talked of little else except the enormity of what we were doing. The more involved we became in our work, the more apparent became our own culpability. We discussed such things as the Nuremberg trials and how they related to our guilt and complicity in the A7D situation. Lawson often expressed his opinion that the brake was downright dangerous and that, once on flight tests, "anything is liable to happen."

I saw his boss, John Warren, at least twice during that month and needled him about what we were doing. He didn't take the jibes too kindly but managed to laugh the situation off as "one of those things." One day I remarked that what we were doing amounted to fraud, and he pulled out an engineering handbook and turned to a section on laws as they related to the engineering profession.

He read the definition of fraud aloud, then said, "Well, technically I don't think what we're doing can be called fraud. I'll admit it's not right, but it's just one of those things. We're just kinda caught in the middle. About all I can tell you is, do like I'm doing. Make copies of everything and put them in your SYA file."

"What's an 'SYA' file?" I asked.

"That's a 'save your ass' file." He laughed.

Although I hadn't known it was called that, I had been keeping an SYA file since the beginning of the A7D fiasco. I had made a copy of every scrap of paper connected even remotely with the A7D and had even had copies of 16 mm movies that had been made during some of the simulated stops. Lawson, too, had an SYA file, and we both maintained them for one reason: Should the true state of events on the A7D ever be questioned, we wanted to have access to a complete set of factual data. We were afraid that should the question ever come up, the test data might accidentally be "lost."

We finished our work on the graphic portion of the report around the first of June. Altogether, we had prepared nearly two hundred pages of data, containing dozens of deliberate falsifications and misrepresentations. I delivered the data to Gretzinger, who said he had been instructed to deliver it personally to the chief engineer, Bud Sunderman, who in turn would assign someone in the engineering department to complete the written portion of the report. He gathered the bundle of data and left the office. Within minutes, he was back with the data, his face white with anger.

"That damned Sink's beat me to it," he said furiously. "He's already talked to Bud about this, and now Sunderman says no one in the engineering department has time to write the report. He wants us to do it, and I told him we couldn't."

The words had barely left his mouth when Russell Line burst in the door. "What the hell's all the fuss about this damned report?" he demanded loudly.

Patiently, Gretzinger explained. "There's no fuss. Sunderman just tole me that we'd have to write the report down here, and I said we couldn't. Russ," he went on, "I've told you before that we weren't going to write the report. I made my position clear on that a long time ago."

Line shut him up with a wave of his hand and, turning to me, bellowed, "I'm getting sick and tired of hearing about this damned report. Now, write the goddam thing and shut up about it!" He slammed out of the office.

Gretzinger and I just sat for a few seconds looking at each other. Then he spoke.

"Well, I guess he's made it pretty clear, hasn't he? We can either write the thing or quit. You know, what we should have done was quiet a long time ago. Now, it's too late."

Somehow, I wasn't at all surprised at this turn of events, and it didn't really make that much difference. As far as I was concerned, we were all up to our necks in the thing anyway, and writing the narrative portion of the report couldn't make me any more guilty than I already felt myself to be.

Still, Line's order came as something of a shock. All the time Lawson and I were working on the report, I felt, deep down, that somewhere, somehow, something would come along and the whole thing would blow over. But Russell Line had crushed that hope. The report was actually going to be issued. Intelligent, law-abiding officials of B. F. Goodrich, one of the oldest and most respected of American corporations, were actually going to deliver to a customer a product that was known to be defective and dangerous and which could very possibly cause death or serious injury.

Within two days, I had completed the narrative, or written portion of the report. As a final sop to my own self-respect, in the conclusion of the report I wrote, "The B. F. Goodrich P/N 2-1162-3 brake assembly does not meet the intent or the requirements of the applicable specification documents and therefore is not qualified."

This was a meaningless gesture, since I knew that this would certainly be changed when the report went through the final typing process. Sure enough, when the report was published, the negative conclusion had been made positive.

One final and significant incident occurred just before publication.

Qualification reports always bear the signature of the person who has prepared them. I refused to sign the report, as did Lawson. Warren was later asked to sign the report. He replied that he would "when I receive a signed statement from Bob Sink ordering me to sign it."

The engineering secretary who was delegated the responsibility of "dogging" the report through publication, told me later that after I, Lawson, and Warren had all refused to sign the report, she had asked Sink if he would sign. He replied, "On something of this nature, I don't think a signature is really needed."

One June 5, 1968, the report was officially published and copies were delivered in person to the Air Force and LTV. Within a week, flight tests were begun at Edwards Air Force Base in California. Searle Lawson was sent to California as Goodrich's representative. Within approximately two weeks, he returned because some rather unusual incidents during the tests had caused them to be canceled.

His face was grim as he related stories of several near crashes during landings—caused by brake troubles. He told me about one incident in which, upon landing, one brake was literally welded together by the intense heat developed during the test stop. The wheel locked, and the plane skidded for nearly 1500 feet before coming to a halt. The plane was jacked up and the wheel removed. The fused parts within the brake had to be pried apart.

Lawson had returned to Troy from California that same day, and that evening, he and others of the Goodrich engineering department left for Dallas for a high-level conference with LTV.

That evening I left work early and went to see my attorney. After I told him the story, he advised that, while I was probably not actually guilty of fraud, I was certainly part of a conspiracy to defraud. He advised me to go to the Federal Bureau of Investigation and offered to arrange an appointment. The following week he took me to the Dayton office of the F.B.I., and after I had been warned that I would not be immune from prosecution, I disclosed the A7D matter to one of the agents. The agent told me to say nothing about the episode to anyone and to report any further incident to him. He said he would forward the story to his superiors in Washington.

A few days later, Lawson returned from the conference in Dallas and said that the Air Force, which had previously approved the qualification report, had suddenly rescinded that approval and was demanding to see some of the raw test data taken during the tests. I gathered that the F.B.I. had passed the word.

Omitting any reference to the F.B.I., I told Lawson I had been to an attorney and that we were probably guilty of conspiracy.

"Can you get me an appointment with your attorney?" he asked. Within a week, he had been to the F.B.I. and told them of his part in the mess. He too was advised to say nothing but to keep on the job reporting any new development.

Naturally, with the rescinding of Air Force approval and the demand to see raw test data, Goodrich officials were in a panic. A conference was called for July 27, a Saturday morning affair at which Lawson, Sink, Warren and myself were present. We met in a tiny conference room in the deserted engineering department. Lawson and I, by now openly hostile to Warren and Sink, ranged ourselves on one side of the conference table while Warren sat on the other side. Sink, chairing the meeting, paced slowly in front of a blackboard, puffing furiously on a pipe.

The meeting was called, Sink began, "to see where we stand on the A7D." What we were going to do, he said, was to "level" with LTV and tell them the "whole truth" about the A7D. "After all," he said, "they're in this thing with us, and they have the right to know how matters stand."

"In other words," I asked, "we're going to tell them the truth?"

"That's right," he replied. "We're going to level with them and let them handle the ball from there."

"There's one thing I don't quite understand," I interjected. "Isn't it going to be pretty hard for us to admit to them that we've lied?"

"Now, wait a minute," he said angrily. "Let's don't go off half-cocked on this thing. It's not a matter of lying. We've just interpreted the information the way we felt it should be."

"I don't know what you call it," I replied, "but to me it's lying, and it's going to be damned hard to confess to them that we've been lying all along."

He became very agitated at this and repeated his "We're not lying," adding, "I don't like this sort of talk."

I dropped the matter at this point, and he began discussing the various discrepancies in the report.

We broke for lunch, and afterward, I came back to the plant to find Sink sitting alone at his desk, waiting to resume the meeting. He called me over and said he wanted to apologize for his outburst that morning. "This thing has kind of gotten me down," he confessed, "and I think you've got the wrong picture. I don't think you really understand everything about this."

Perhaps so, I conceded, but it seemed to me that if we had already told LTV one thing and then had to tell them another, changing our story completely, we would have to admit we were lying.

"No," he explained patiently, "we're not really lying. All we were doing was interpreting the figures the way we knew they should be. We were just exercising engineering license."

During the afternoon session, we marked some forty-three discrepant points in the report: forty-three points that LTV would surely spot as occasions where we had exercised "engineering license."

After Sink listed those points on the blackboard, we discussed each one individually. As each point came up, Sink would explain that it was probably "too minor to bother about," or that perhaps it "wouldn't be wise to open that can of worms," or that maybe this was a point that "LTV just wouldn't understand." When the meeting was over, it had been decided that only three points were "worth mentioning."

Similar conferences were held during August and September, and the summer was punctuated with frequent treks between Dallas and Troy, and demands by the Air Force to see the raw test data. Tempers were short and matters seemed to grow worse.

Finally, early in October 1968, Lawson submitted his resignation, to take effect on October 25. On October 18, I submitted my own resignation, to take effect on November 1. In my resignation, addressed to Russell Line, I cited the A7D report and stated: "As you are aware, this report contained numerous deliberate and willful misrepresentations which, according to legal counsel, constitute fraud and expose both myself and others to criminal charges of conspiracy to defraud. . . . The events of the past seven months have created an atmosphere of deceit and distrust in which it is impossible to work. . . ."

On October 25, I received a sharp summons to the office of Bud Sunderman. As chief engineer at the Troy plant, Sunderman was responsible for the entire engineering division. Tall and graying, impeccably dressed at all times, he was capable of producing a dazzling smile or a hearty chuckle or immobilizing his face into marble hardness, as the occasion required.

I faced the marble hardness when I reached his office. He motioned me to a chair. "I have your resignation here," he snapped, "and I must say you have made some rather shocking, I might even say irresponsible, charges. This is very serious."

Before I could reply, he was demanding an explanation. "I want to know exactly what the fraud is in connection with the A7D and how you can dare accuse this company of such a thing!"

I started to tell some of the things that had happened during the testing, but he shut me off saying, "There's nothing wrong with anything we've done here. You aren't aware of all the things that have been going on behind the scenes. If you had known the true situation, you would never have made these charges." He said that in view of my apparent "disloyalty" he had decided to accept my resignation "right now," and said it would be better for all concerned if I left the plant immediately. As I got up to leave he asked me if I intended to "carry this thing further."

I answered simply, "Yes," to which he replied, "Suit yourself." Within twenty minutes, I had cleaned out my desk and left. Forty-eight hours later, the B. F. Goodrich Company recalled the qualification report and the four-disk brake, announcing that it would replace the brake with a new, improved, five-disk brake at no cost to LTV.

Ten months later, on August 13, 1969, I was the chief government witness at a hearing conducted before Senator William Proxmire's Economy in Government Subcommittee of the Congress's Joint Economic Committee. I related the A7D story to the committee, and my testimony was supported by Searle Lawson, who followed me to the witness stand. Air Force officers also testified, as well as a four-man team from the General Accounting Office, which had conducted an investigation of the A7D brake at the request of Senator Proxmire. Both Air Force and GAO investigators declared that the brake was dangerous and had not been tested properly.

Testifying for Goodrich was R. G. Jeter, vice-president and general counsel of the company, from the Akron headquarters. Representing the Troy plant was Robert Sink. These two denied any wrongdoing on the part of the Goodrich Company, despite expert testimony to the contrary by Air Force and GAO officials. Sink was quick to deny any connection with the writing of the report or of directing any falsifications, claiming to be on the West Coast at the time. John Warren was the man who supervised its writing, said Sink.

As for me, I was dismissed as a high-school graduate with no technical training, while Sink testified that Lawson was a young, inexperienced engineer. "We tried to give him guidance," Sink testified, "but he preferred to have his own convictions."

About changing the data and figures in the report, Sink said: "When you take data from several different sources, you have to rationalize among those data what is the true story. This is part of your engineering know-how." He admitted that changes had been made in the data, "but only to make them more consistent with the over-all picture of the data that is available."

Jeter pooh-poohed the suggestion that anything improper occurred, saying: "We have thirty-odd engineers at this plant . . . and I say to you that it is incredible that these men would stand idly by and see reports changed or falsified. . . . I mean you just do not have to do that working for anybody. . . . Just nobody does that."

The four-hour hearing adjourned with no real conclusion reached by the committee. But, the following day the Department of Defense made sweeping changes in its inspection, testing and reporting procedures. A spokesman for the DOD said that changes were a result of the Goodrich episode.

The A7D is now in service, sporting a Goodrich-made five-disk brake, a brake that works very well, I'm told. Business at the Goodrich plant is good. Lawson is now an engineer for LTV and has been assigned to the A7D project. And I am now a newspaper reporter.

At this writing [1972], those remaining at Goodrich are still secure in the same positions, all except Russell Line and Robert Sink. Line has been rewarded with a promotion to production superintendent, a large step upward on the corporate ladder. As for Sink, he moved up into Line's old job.

13 / Benton Harlow: Distributor of Unsafe Drugs

JAMES T. CAREY

THE FOLLOWING is a shortened version of an interview conducted with a former executive of a drug company in the Midwest, a subsidiary of a national parent corporation. He and several of his colleagues, were convicted of lying to the Food and Drug Administration about animal studies testing the effects of an antichloesterol drug developed by the company, and of fraud in responding to reports that the drug casued cataracts in the eyes of rats. The grand jury that indicted these three officers also returned a twelve-count indictment against the company and its parent organization. The subsidiary pleaded no contest to six counts and the senior corporation to two. The subsidiary was fined $60,000 and the parent enterprise $20,000. All three corporate officers indicted also pleaded guilty to six counts. At the time of the interview Mr. Harlow was in his early 60s and living in retirement. He was sentenced to six months probation and retired several years after his conviction because he felt his own opportunities to move ahead had vanished. The city within which he was born and worked was dominated by his drug firm and a large soap manufacturer. The executives of both companies were charter members of the city's business elite. Harlow was educated at a church-related liberal arts college and went on to get a master's degree in business administration. His first position after leaving school was in sales at a competing drug firm. He was recruited for his next company, the one from which he retired, seven years later.

Question: Let's start by your telling me some of the circumstances surrounding the controversial drug HE/14.

Harlow: Well, in the early 1950s there was a tremendous push to develop a drug that would be effective in treating heart disease. The public was clamoring for something espe-

163

cially since they were convinced that cholesterol was the culprit. So we began experimenting with a variety of compounds to reduce the body's cholesterol levels. That's how we developed HE/14. It was developed here in our own laboratories. It's one of a number of compounds that fall under the generic name of triparanol.

Question: What is the usual procedure when a drug like that has been developed? How do you find out if it's effective or not?

Harlow: We began a series of tests on rats, monkeys, and dogs and sent the results of those tests to the Food and Drug Administration. The tests showed that HE/14 reduced the cholesterol or inhibited its functions in lower animals. In our application to market the drug we had to show that it was safe for laboratory animals and had no serious side effects when taken with humans. They changed those regulations a few years later so that now you have to demonstrate a drug's effectiveness as well.

Question: Was there considerable enthusiasm in the company for the new drug?

Harlow: Oh, definitely. We thought we really had something. As you may know the drug industry is tremendously competitive and even if your market position is strong you can't stand still for long. We were hoping that HE/14 would be a shot in the arm for us, reinforce our position in the industry and bring in more money to finance our plans for expansion. We thought this would be the drug that would help us break into the big time.

Question: Was there any concern within the company that the drug's introduction should be delayed until further tests were made to see if there were any negative side effects?

Harlow: Well, this is something that was stressed by the government prosecutor but all I can say is that we thought we were operating in an unknown area where the risks were high and we knew our competitors were also working on the same kind of thing. It just would have been foolhardy to delay until further tests were made. When do you stop making tests? You can always be criticized for not going further no matter how much testing you do. We had faith in what we were doing and we thought we could save many lives with HE/14.

Question: As I recall the FDA did not approve your application immediately but asked for further test data. Can you tell me a little more about that?

Harlow: That's the role FDA is supposed to play. They move cautiously and some of their scientists are very suspicious of the drug industry. Our own scientists feel that the FDA group is basically obstructionist. They seem to get some secret pleasure out of blocking potentially useful drugs. The pharmacologists there are not very well respected in the industry.

Question: Why is that?

Harlow: They aren't very competent. If they were, they'd be working somewhere else. Also they seem very responsive to political pressure. That's what we thought was happening with the delay on our initial application. So we mounted a promotional campaign to persuade them. We asked physicians to try the drug on their private patients and report their results to us. I wasn't connected with that operation so I don't know how successful it was. But in 1960 the FDA approved our application with the condition that we list some side effects.

Question: What were the side effects?

Harlow: They had received scattered reports on vomiting, nausea, and dermatitis. So we put that on the label as possible side effects and started selling it.

Question: Let's back up a little to the test results you sent in originally. Were there any problems with those?

Harlow: The government made much of the fact that they were supposed to have been falsified. They relied mainly on a former disgruntled employee who claimed that what she recorded in her own laboratory book was left out in the original application. As a result of her complaint the FDA sent a team to look at our records and interview lab employees. The government claimed that the lab director instructed his assistants to revise their data. I think they put the wrong construction of this whole series of early tests. I'm not a pharmacologist but I do know that you have to rework laboratory data and summarize it concisely so it's understandable to a lay audience. All drug laboratories do this, it's called "smoothing out the data." It isn't falsification.

Question: Was the drug called off the market after the FDA team looked at your laboratories and records?

Harlow: No, not then, but there was a campaign developing against HE/14 which wasn't quite as disinterested as the FDA made it out to be. For instance our major competitor was encouraged to test our version of triparanol with its own anticholesterol drug which they were preparing to market.

Question: What did they find?

Harlow: Just what you'd expect—that HE/14 had negative side effects that their own compound didn't.

Question: Did they list any side effects that you hadn't included on your label?

Harlow: Yes, they said their animals developed cataracts and started losing their hair.

Question: What was the reaction within your company to this report?

Harlow: Some of us were beginning to have questions about the side effects. But we couldn't be sure it was related to HE/14 or something else. You can never know with absolute certainty. So we felt we had to go ahead and defend our product.

Question: Was there ever any discussion about the ethics of the situation?

Harlow: If you mean did we think we were unethical, absolutely not. The government accused us of being criminals. That upset me very much. I have always thought of myself as a law-abiding person. If it turned out that the negative side effects were due to something other than HE/14, then we would have been applauded for having stood up to the FDA. It's happened in other instances. I have a history of heart disease and I was taking HE/14 myself right up till the time it was withdrawn. I know several other executives here were also. That doesn't sound very criminal to me.

Question: In your internal company discussions were there any suggestions that the drug should be withdrawn for safety reasons?

Harlow: I don't recall that there were. If anyone felt that way privately it was not expressed. Our initial decision to go with HE/14 and all the investment of time, effort and money we put into it—well, we just couldn't back down. Even after it was withdrawn we still had a $2 million inventory of HE/14. How were we supposed to absorb that loss?

Question: I take it you think the action of the Justice Department in proceeding against you was unfair?

Harlow: Yes, I do—terribly unfair. If they're saying what we did was wrong, then I don't know what they're suggesting. What would you have done in a similar situation? If you don't have firms competing with each other to develop new miracle drugs, then you've got stagnation. Maybe that's what the FDA wants—complete control over developing and testing new drugs and selling them. That would mean the end of the drug industry.

Question: What was the reaction within the company to your conviction?

Harlow: It was expected and they knew someone had to take responsibility. If I refused then my case as well as a score of others would have gone to trial, which could have been disastrous both for me personally and the company. The judge in his remarks on sentencing held the company responsible. He said it was a failure of executive, managerial, and supervisional control. But the amount the company was fined was ridiculous.

Question: So the reaction of your colleagues was that you sacrificed yourself for the organization?

Harlow: Yes, but it wasn't that strong and it didn't last very long. I was given a substantial raise the following year but from then on my responsibilities were gradually shifted to others. I saw what was happening and requested retirement. They were quite generous—I'm on full salary now until I'm 65 and then will start drawing my retirement benefits.

Discussion

There was a uncanny similarity between Mr. Harlow's background and those of the convicted electrical industry conspirators. He was somewhat older at the time of his conviction but he was making well over $100,000 a year. He graduated from a prestigious liberal arts college and received a master's degree from a nationally recognized school of business administration. He was married, the father of two grown children, and had been an officer in the U. S. Army during World War II. He was active on a variety of boards and committees in his home community, including the YMCA, Chamber of Commerce, United Community Fund, and, ironically, Big Brothers. He was quite active in local fund-raising activities for the Presbyterian Church. He had no previous arrests.

The differential association explanation seems compatible with Harlow's account. He did not report any extensive discussion of the position the company was to take. Everybody seemed to agree on the course of action that should be followed. Harlow expressed some surprise that what he considered acceptable practice was viewed by the Justice Department as illegal. It was perhaps this unanimity among the executives about the appropriateness of their action that accounts for Harlow's surprise at the Justice Department's reaction. No one involved expressed any strong repugnance or even opposition to selling the unsafe drug. Rather they all seemed to drift into the activity without thinking a great deal about it. If anyone was opposed to the company's position, they didn't make their opposition known. Harlow saw the activity as necessary, though risky, and basic to his company's survival. He believed the activity was generated by the intense competition among drug firms. One conclusion that is implied in this account is that cutthroat competition does not insure product safety, at least in areas where the danger of the product is not immediately apparent.

The gradual building of commitment to marketing the drug was not recounted in much detail but it seems clear that there were a number of "side bets" . . . that gave consistency to the plan of action that finally emerged. Harlow spoke of the investment of time, effort, and money put into it that precluded any backing out. An appellate court judge ruling on a later damages claim against the company also commented on this process: "some weight must be given to the human tendency to follow a course of conduct once decided upon even when considerations have appeared that would have led to a different decision at the outset, a tendency particularly strong when large investments of both effort and money have been made; the very fact of the initial decision importantly affects subsequent ones."

Harlow did not think of himself as a criminal. At most he would argue that what he did was technically illegal. In this his attitude paralleled those of the electrical conspirators. One General Electric vice-president stated before going to jail:

> All of you know that next Monday, in Philadelphia, I will start serving a thirty-day jail term, along with six other *businessmen* for conduct which has been *interpreted* as being in conflict with *complex* antitrust laws.

Even though his sentence of six months' probation was minimal it had a pronounced psychological impact on Harlow. The possibilities of a jail sentence seemed quite frightening, underlining the sensitivity of corporate offenders like Harlow to status deprivation and censure. The fact that violations carry criminal penalties addresses head on the tendency of corporate offenders to rationalize them. In this they are much like the shoplifters Cameron studied:

> Again and again store people explain to pilferers that they are under arrest as thieves, that they will, in the normal course of events, be taken in a police van to jail, held in jail until bond is raised, and tried in court before a judge and sentenced. Interrogation procedures at the store are directed specifically and consciously toward breaking down any illusion that the shoplifter may possess that his behavior is merely regarded as "naughty" or "bad." . . . It becomes increasingly clear to the pilferer that he is considered a thief and is in imminent danger of being hauled into court and publicly exhibited as such. This realization is often accompanied by dramatic changes in attitudes and by severe emotional disturbance.

Harlow's justifications fit in with his self-image as a law-abiding person but these were shaken by his conviction. He saw nothing wrong with his identification with the company and its concern with healing the sick, its zeal for producing efficient effective drugs at low cost. The extent of his confidence is revealed by the fact that he took HE/14 for his own heart condition right up until it was removed from the market, though he had more reasons to question it than the hapless salesmen who distributed it.

The seriousness of the violations was never recognized by the company itself. Their philosophy was that the violations were part and parcel of the hazards inherent in discovering and marketing new drugs. A number of civil damage suits were brought against the company even though criminal trial records were not available as evidence. The reports on the effect of the drug were frightening: cataracts, loss of hair, painful dryness of the skin, and other complications. The impact of the fine on the company was trifling. One year after the fine, the company increased its profits by more than 10 percent—more than enough to cover the $60,000 fine imposed, the maximum limit possible under the law. Harlow thought that the fine was ridiculous and that its deterrent effect was nil. Presumably a larger fine or perhaps the requirement that all illegal profits from the sale of HE/14 be disgorged would bring home the lesson more forcefully. The one option the court had to deal more severely with the company was to reject their pleas of *nolo contendere*. This the judge chose not to do, thus making damages of claims against the company more difficult to sustain. Sutherland's original notions about corporate crime are substantiated in this case: the courts dealt sympathetically with all the violators and the news media covered the case briefly under "business news." The company had no training program to alert its executives to the legal hazards of what they were doing. Perhaps if that were a condition of the company's "probation," future violations would be less likely.

The company's response to Harlow's conviction also reveals their attitude toward the violations. He was given a substantial raise following the conviction and encouraged to resign before 65. Some of the electrical conspirators were fired by their companies, others were rewarded. There seemed to be some recognition that Harlow had performed a service for the company, but also some embarrassment at keeping him around any longer than necessary.

Harlow's comments on the way new drugs are marketed and his negative views of FDA attempts to regulate it suggest that the industry itself is criminogenic. There are few built-in safeguards to insure that the health and safety of potential consumers would be protected. The violations that occurred in the drug industry—as well as those in the electrical industry, milk and bread industry, plumbing, and other major industries—took place in a context where success, greater profits, and enlarging the company's market took precedence over all other values. . . .

14 / Exposing Risks of Nuclear Disaster [Confessions of a Whistle Blower]

PETER FAULKNER

In 1974 I was working for the Nuclear Services Corporation (NSC) as a systems application engineer when, through my studies of safety, management, and reliability problems, I became aware of many engineering deficiencies in nuclear power systems that were already on the market. After a period of indecision about keeping this information to myself and not jeopardizing my career, I began to draft a paper critical of the commercial nuclear industry. On March 12, 1974, I presented this paper to a U.S. Senate subcommittee. Three weeks later, I was fired from my job. I then forwarded to several government agencies copies of confidential, proprietary industry documents, owned by the Edison Electric Institute (EEI), that confirmed many of the mechanical problems and design inadequacies in nuclear power systems I identified in my Senate paper. I also released confidential memoranda by Paul Dragoumis, then vice-president of the Potomac Electric Power Company's (PEPCO) nuclear engineering and construction group, who identified potentially dangerous design defects in General Electric reactor containments.

As I expected, my engineering career ended abruptly. None of these acts would have been necessary if design inadequacies and defects had been fewer or less severe, or if government and industry had devoted primary efforts toward solving them instead of promoting nuclear technology. I decided that they were necessary in 1974 because public safety was being compromised by the nuclear industry and I am still of this opinion. This conviction compelled me to warn other citizens and the federal government about industry problems.

When the government failed to take action I began to realize that, instead of being part of the solution, it was part of the problem.

Shortly afterwards, the industry succeeded to some extent in suppressing the charges and documentary evidence I had tried to bring forward. The government took no action regarding my Senate paper and the controversy died down for awhile. However, other engineers and scientists have since made similar accusations and the industry is now suffering the consequences. Specifically, several plants were shut down, most notably Humboldt Bay, Indian Point One, and Dresden One, and others have experienced extended outages; construction and operating permits have been delayed indefinitely; and the industry's worst accident to date—the March 1979 partial meltdown at the Three Mile Island (TMI) nuclear plant—has seriously undermined public confidence in nuclear power. Seven months later, the Report of the President's Commission on the Accident (also know as the Kemeny Commission Report) concluded that the TMI plant was not equipped with adequate safety apparatus, its operators were poorly trained, its emergency procedures were defective, and its control room was not set up to cope with a major emergency. The Commission found that the Nuclear Regulatory Commission (NRC), when called upon to manage the crisis, performed with "marked ineptitude." The Report's summary judgment was: "With its present organization, staff and attitudes, the NRC is unable to fulfill its responsibility for providing an acceptable level of safety for a nuclear power plant." Unfortunately, there are many nuclear plants with problems similar to TMI's and the government's difficulties in coping with the emergency is symptomatic of several deeper problems.

My concern regarding the legitimacy of nuclear power reached a peak more than five years before the TMI accident. This concern arose from firsthand experience at five nuclear plants where I served as a consulting engineer. By the time I was assigned to PEPCO in late 1973, I began to realize the extent to which many safety and reliability problems in nuclear systems derived from overconfident engineering, the failure to test nuclear systems fully in intermediate stages, and competitive pressures that forced reactor manufacturers to market their systems before serious design problems were resolved. (The industry's standard practice was "sell first, test later.") A case in point involved General Electric's (GE) Mark III containment design concept. The Paul Dragoumis memoranda mentioned earlier described three serious design problems in the Mark III system that were still under negotiation two years after the concept was released for marketing. The design problems raised serious questions about the integrity of General Electric's entire product line. I was concerned that a reasonable doubt existed about the safety of over 40 plants in and outside of the United States. In particular, I was worried that workers at the communities near power stations using the Mark III containment might suffer unreasonable risk of radiation exposure. Gradually, I came to realize that a combination of greed and poor planning by government and industry caused unacceptable delays in essential reactor prototype tests. One result of these delays was that the upgrading of safety standards came too late to benefit plants already built. In other cases, plants under construction or on line had to be redesigned; often, expensive components or entire systems had to be torn down and rebuilt. Some deficiencies did not become known until plants were already operating.

Just as I was beginning to doubt the adequacy of the industry's safety controls, I also came to realize that both employer and client expected me to keep these doubts to myself, despite documentary evidence. The rationale for doing so seemed reasonable at the time. The industry was just beginning to mature; plants had not been on line long enough to provide enough data for harsh judgments; bugs were being worked out; and nuclear industry people were learning as they went along. In short, everyone seemed to be doing the best job possible under the circumstances. Why should I take the chance of throwing away my engineering career in a promising field?

There were many reasons why I decided to "blow the whistle" on my employers and the industry as a whole. First, electric generation by nuclear fission involves a technology with an unprecedented capacity for environmental and human damage. Second, I was convinced that there really was a better way to build nuclear plants and that third-party inspection of systems and components—essential to their safe operation—was conspicuously missing from the nuclear industry's quality assurance programs. Third, I was sure that if I presented my criticisms to several agencies at once, I would get a fair hearing; my proposals would not be covered up, and I would either force the industry to implement some long-overdue reforms or would convince the public that the industry was so badly managed that a major reactor accident was imminent. Finally, and most important, I had overwhelming evidence that many nuclear systems were sold before they were properly designed—a practice that carried these systems through the entire construction phase, and sometimes into operation, with unresolved technical questions.

I spoke to many of my fellow engineers and shared their observations and opinions on the industry in an attempt to be sure that I was not merely being a gadfly and that I was indeed defining the problem properly and raising pertinent questions. But although many of my colleagues with far more civilian nuclear experience than I were well aware of the abysmal industry management, I began to realize that they had no desire to "rock the boat." They moved from one day to the next with a benign optimism. The general feeling was that the industry eventually would solve most of these problems and that line engineers should leave complex management and policy problems to executives and experts. It began to appear that I was working with people who had long since accepted their roles as narrow specialists; this perception allowed them to shrug off any responsibility for nuclear industry management problems, even though they saw more clearly than most the hazards posed by inadequate design and testing. Meanwhile, the industry was suffering chronic delays and shutdowns, which created a potentially infinite demand for our services as consulting engineers. I found the inherent conflict of interest intolerable; the awesome safety implications demanded that someone identify and propose solutions for management deficiencies, even though doing so might eliminate future demand for his services.

A small group of us designed a pilot management information system to secure a better degree of quality assurance for our clients and to consider management problems at a deeper level. When this was rejected and when I was told by several senior engineers that our clients didn't want management advice—only technical assistance to get them over the next hill—it occurred to me that no one wanted to explore or remedy the underlying problems.

Late in 1973, I asked my superior, Dr. Harry Lawroski, NSC's environmental systems manager and then treasurer of the American Nuclear Society, to help me prepare a paper for publication by the Institute of Environmental Sciences (IES). The paper's abstract emphasized that the nuclear industry had allowed its management philosophy to lag behind its technical development and it proposed centralizing certain functions such as contract negotiation and quality assurance enforcement. Dr. Lawroski approved the abstract in October 1973, and IES accepted it. The initial draft was developed on my own time in November, after I had been assigned by NSC to the Potomac Electric Power Company in Washington, D.C., to assist Paul Dragoumis and Russell Brown with developing PEPCO's comprehensive quality assurance/management information system for the Douglas Point nuclear station.

Two weeks after arriving in Washington, I contacted John Tunney, who at the time was a Senator from California and also a friend from my college and Air Force days. Before running for Congress, John had been my personal attorney, but this time I was the one who was offering advice. I warned John that he should familiarize himself with nuclear industry problems, since they would soon be potent political issues, and I indicated that I would be gald to give him my views. John invited me to meet with two of his assistants, Dan Jaffe and Bob Feyer. Several meetings later, I started work on a background briefing memo for John based on the IES paper, then in its third draft.

Although both papers recommended reforms, I was beginning to wonder if the real problem was with the people in the nuclear industry. There did not seem to be enough really first-rate engineers and executives like Dragoumis and his staff. I had come to respect them immensely, especially when compared with personnel at other electric power companies. If indeed there was a shortage of able people in the industry, it was unlikely that a few legislative or administrative changes would make much difference. And since large numbers of first-rate technical and management people obviously could not be drafted en masse, perhaps my friends at NSC were right in ignoring what they could not change.

Although I couldn't determine the quality of engineer-executives in the nuclear industry without spending years visiting every U.S. electric power company and related federal agency, I had, by this time, gathered plenty of subjective data on management and technical adequacy. But I did not act on this data until similar allegations by Louis Roddis, then vice chairman of the board of Consolidated Edison of New York, confirmed my suspicions.

Roddis was a 1937 graduate of the U.S. Naval Academy who had a distinguished career in the Navy, including an appointment by Admiral Hyman Rickover as one of the first site engineers in the nuclear submarine program. After leaving the Navy, Roddis joined Con Ed and became its president while the first nuclear plants in New York— Indian Point Units 1 and 2—were under construction. Roddis showed special concern for issues involving safety, design integrity, and the hazards of balancing investment return against high engineering standards. In November 1972, he made an astonishing speech before the Atomic Industrial Forum (AIF), of which he was president, entitled "Maintaining the Output, or Can We Get There from Here?" Roddis submitted data that nuclear plants were generating electricity at a rate of 20 percent less than what had been promised earlier in environmental impact statements. He called for several reforms and, judging by industry reactions, upset a number of people. Industry observers believe that the AIF speech contributed to forces that "promoted" him to his 1973–74 position—more honorary than functional—of vice chairman of the Con Ed board of directors.

On February 3, 1974, the New York *Times* published a short article based on an interview with Roddis, nearly 17 months after his AIF speech. Roddis repeated his earlier charges and alleged that spot checks of plant performance convinced him that nuclear plant electricity production was still far below expectations. He accused industry executives of publishing misleading plant performance data that depicted nuclear plants as producing far more electricity than they really were. Roddis seemed to be telling the industry that it was being doubly dishonest with the public—in its attempts to refute his own earlier data and conclusions, and in trying to foster citizen support for nuclear power by using irrelevant data that concealed the real state of affairs.

Convinced of Roddis's honesty, I was sure that he would make these allegations a second time only if he were under fire and furious about it. After reading the *Times* article and obtaining a copy of Roddis's 1972 speech, I checked his data and decided that he was right. If the industry was putting pressure on him to recant his earlier conclusions, I had good reason to question the industry leaders' ethics, as well as their managerial and technical competence.

The last part of the puzzle fell into place a few days later. It was on February 10, 1974, while I was working at PEPCO, that I happened to pick up a copy of a memo, written by Paul Dragoumis, from the PEPCO project manager's desk. It described negotiations between his staff and GE on several serious design problems evident in the billion-dollar Mark III system he had purchased from GE. The most stunning comment in the memo was: "The design of many contemporary containments, not just Mark III, may be in substantial question."

Paul Dragoumis was no ordinary engineer, and this memorandum, containing complete documentation, gave me special cause for alarm. A fiercely aggressive and technically brilliant young executive (he was then 37) with a leading U.S. power company, Dragoumis was without a doubt one of the nuclear industry's best and brightest. Certainly, such a man would be in line for the presidency of the American Nuclear Society, an electric power company, or both. The memos represented Dragoumis's best judgment on design problems that were not resolved before GE released its design concept for marketing. GE apparently gambled that it could market the Mark III, that all technical problems were solvable, and that all would be ironed out in later negotiations between GE and its customers.

I decided soon after that the public should know about this and that I would distribute copies of Dragoumis's memos without his knowledge or permission. If Dragoumis was right, then public safety took precedence over all other considerations—his career and mine, PEPCO's plans to build a plant, industry profits, and adequate electric supply for the country. For what his memos showed beyond a doubt were that serious design defects existed in GE's product line and that GE had rushed its containment design to market before any large-scale prototype tests were run. This amounted to a serious breach of engineering ethics. It also obliged purchasers to become involved in the testing phase, including design verification, prototype, data analysis and, in this case, redesign of the initial concept. The ethics breach turned on the fact that this involvement also imposed a difficult dilemma as well as potential financial losses on purchasers of GE systems if any of these postponed tests yielded problems too difficult to solve. For if any of these problems—Anticipated Transient Without SCRAM (ATWS), for example—were identified as essentially unsolvable after hundreds of millions of dollars were invested, fiscal considerations would weigh heavily in any decision to shut down the project. The momentum at that point would favor going ahead and accepting the risk.

My decision to leak Dragoumis's memos reflected a personal value judgment that, in view of the enormous health hazard, this method of dealing with risks was not acceptable, that it had been going on for years in the nuclear industry, and that it was time to put a stop to it by selective surgery at the point where risks were metastasizing throughout the design and construction cycles.

At this point I stopped giving the industry that employed me the benefit of the doubt. A great many things that bothered me for months began to fall into place: co-workers' comments that power company management was more often than not either incompetent or unequal to the job of running nuclear plants; the suggestion that electric power company top brass had no idea how different, how much more complex, nuclear plants were compared to fossil-fueled plants. Roddis's implied charge that the industry was cutting corners trying to get nuclear plants sold, licensed, and running at any cost confirmed my interpretation of Dragoumis's report that adequate prototype testing was being conducted *after* nuclear systems were marketed. In the end, Roddis's allegations reinforced and integrated all these fragments into one consistent view. Instead of minimizing their significance, I began to seek confirmation and other evidence of dishonesty and incompetence elsewhere in the industry.

At the same time, I completely rewrote both the Tunney and IES papers, spotlighting Roddis's data as the basis for questioning plant safety and reliability, and, ultimately, the competence of industry leaders. In the papers I discussed Rossis's finding that nuclear plants are generating almost 20 percent less electricity than industry executives promised when they applied for hundreds of construction permits between 1966 and 1972. This meant that, if these electric generation rates continued, it would be necessary to build 20 percent more plants to obtain the amount of electric generating capacity promised earlier. The 20 percent shortfall also indicated to me that safety and reliability were less than adequate.

I also mentioned in the papers that frequent and unexpected breakdowns in plant systems have caused unsatisfactory electricity production. Nuclear plants are breaking down frequently and unexpectedly because they are not built properly in the first place—that goes for plant design, procurement, fabrication, construction, and testing. The most effective guarantee that a plant will be built and operated properly is a rigorous quality assurance program implemented from the earliest design stages throughout the years of plant operation. Quality assurance (QA) during these phases of nuclear plant development is inadequate for a great many reasons. For example, third-party inspection of components and systems is not required. Also, nuclear plant management and staff regard QA with resignation and suspicion. But since quality assurance is required by the federal government, many electric power companies reluctantly go through the motions of hiring outside firms like NSC to write their quality assurance programs, appointing marginal engineers from their own staffs to implement them.

I finished the final drafts of the Tunney and IES papers in mid-February. I then forwarded the IES draft to the Institute for comment and delivered the Tunney paper personally to Bob Feyer. On February 25, he called to thank me and to mention that the Senator did not plan any immediate action. Later, I learned that any senator or congressman proposing legislative reforms based on my paper would have embroiled himself in the type of controversy that could seriously damage a political career. Rather than commiserate with John, I forwarded a copy of my paper to Anthony Z. Roisman, a prominent Washington attorney, who urged me to allow him to include it in the U.S. Senate proceedings. I agreed.

At the end of February I returned to California briefly and showed the IES draft to my superiors. Dr. Lawroski thought it was too strong and told me to rewrite it. On March 6, I flew back to Washington to resume my engineering duties at PEPCO and to wait for Roisman to make his move.

By this time my own position had hardened. What started as a technical paper recommending legislative and management reforms became a deliberate attempt to challenge the nuclear industry from within. I had decided to test Roddis's argument and data by resubmitting them to the public. I wanted to know who pressured him and how they made him angry enough to accuse his colleagues of dishonesty. One way to find out was to publicize a paper using his data—adding my own arguments—and to see if the same thing happened to me. I wanted to find out if the nuclear industry was as dishonest and manipulative as Roddis claimed.

On March 12, 1974, a slightly revised version of the Tunney paper was read into the Senate subcommittee Energy Research and Development Administration hearings record by Tony Roisman. On March 15, my lead engineer recalled me from Washington and explained that several power company executives had telephoned Sherman Naymark, NSC's president, to complain about my Senate paper.

On March 18, I returned to the California home office and met with Naymark. I admitted to having forwarded drafts of the IES paper to the Institute, but pointed out that circulating drafts for comment and officially publishing a paper were two different things. If the data or reasoning seemed to warrant revision, I would change the draft before publication. I also admitted forwarding the other paper to Tunney, with a copy to Roisman. I insisted that the writing of what eventually became the Senate paper, revising it to include Roddis's data, and instructing Roisman to submit it to the Senate committee were acts of a *private citizen,* not those of an employee of NSC.

Naymark argued that I acquired my nuclear industry information while gaining experience as an NSC employee, that the paper was directly related to NSC activities, and that I had been identified by the complaining executives as an employee of NSC. I protested that these executives were defining my authorship differently than I intended and that instead of pressuring my employer, they should have gotten in touch with me personally. I asked who applied pressure on NSC and Naymark told me that Southern California Edison and Northern States Power Company, as well as about ten others, phoned him.

Naymark expressed extreme concern about the Senate paper and became quite upset when I mentioned that I hoped to forward copies of it to other agencies. He led me to believe that if I showed "good faith" by withdrawing the IES paper from publication, he would be grateful. The implication was that pressure on me would cease. I did not realize at the time that he was setting me up for termination. I reluctantly withdrew the IES paper, believing that it would be impossible to get anything approaching what I wanted to say cleared by NSC.

On March 23, Dr. John Turner, NSC's company psychiatrist, interrogated me for four hours. His questions attempted to determine whether some hidden motivations or deep-seated hostility on my part were the basis "for circulating papers that you must have known would be embarrassing to NSC." I replied that this was a simple case of citizen duty transcending personal or employee commitments. On Monday, March 25, I retained Michael Kennedy as my attorney. Early the following week, on April 2, 1974, Naymark fired me on the grounds that my usefulness to the company had ended.

After my dismissal, I sent copies of my Senate paper to the New York *Times,* the *Christian Science Monitor,* several New York investment banking firms, Ralph Nader, the California State Public Utilities Commission, and various senators and congressmen. To bolster my argument, I added copies of a lengthy collection of operating reports from all nuclear plants in the U.S.—gathered by the EEI Prime Movers Committee—and copies of the Dragoumis memoranda, which I copied while at PEPCO. There were several documents of an even more sensitive nature that I withheld and stored in safe deposit boxes. I notified industry leaders that if anything happened to me, my attorney would call a press conference and release them.

I then notified the FBI that after I had voluntarily made my views available to a U.S. Senate subcommittee and I was fired from my job barely three weeks later. This, I told the Bureau, was a violation of Title 18, Section 1505 of the U.S. Code, which protects congressional witnesses from reprisal. Keith Barry of the San Jose FBI office initiated a preliminary investigation. In August 1975, the Department of Justice, alleging that I had not been subpoenaed, instructed Barry to end his investigation. I pointed out to him that the precedent set by the disposition of my case appeared to deny statutory immunity to voluntary witnesses who come forward with important information bearing on public safety. Barry said that I was not protected by the law because I had not appeared physically before the subcommittee but, instead, presented the Senate paper through a third party. I told him that I thought this should make no difference, that the same immunities should apply. I maintained that the only relevant facts were that I presented my views openly and voluntarily, that they were accepted and published in the Senate record, and that I was fired soon after. I felt that immunities were being denied to me on very narrow, technical grounds and that the Department of Justice displayed a curious unwillingness to pursue the matter—an unwillingness that, in my opinion, may have resulted from pressure by the nuclear industry.

While the Department of Justice was considering termination of Barry's investigation in April 1975, the Nuclear Regulatory Commission (NRC) announced one of a different sort—not by an independent agency, but by General Electric's customers and by GE itself into the adequacy of its containment system. The Commission explained that the investigation was triggered by "new" data which related to "previously unidentified" hydrodynamic forces that could develop during reactor operation. Dragoumis's memos show that General Electric learned for the first time about these problems on or before

June 1973, and *not* the spring of 1975 as the NRC announcement implies. The memos also confirm that GE explicitly minimized the significance of these problems until prototype tests—delayed more than 18 months after the system was released for marketing—showed that these forces could jeopardize nuclear reactor safety.

The 1975 NRC announcement affected 16 electric power companies with 25 General Electric reactors, and required a thorough review of the design adequacy of these plants on the basis that some twenty dynamic loading conditions were ignored in the original design. These same conditions existed to some degree in all other General Electric containments under negotiation, construction, or fabrication. The potential costs to the power companies and ratepayers for correcting containment deficiencies are substantial. The containment system itself is simply not replaceable with a new and improved model; it forms the envelope surrounding the nuclear steam supply system and thereby is inextricably involved with many other vital systems and structures.

Shortly after the NRC announcement, General Electric appointed Dale Bridenbaugh as manager of the Mark I containment review team. Over a period of months, Dale and two other GE engineers, Greg Minor and Dick Hubbard, considered the serious safety questions that were beginning to emerge. In February 1976, all three of them resigned their jobs and began a series of appearances to educate Congress and the public about nuclear risks. The detailed congressional testimony of the "GE Three" tends to confirm my interpretation of the Dragoumis memos and several allegations regarding inadequate quality assurance that appear in my Senate paper.

Since April 1974, I have applied to sixty-seven U.S. corporations for employment in technical areas. All applications have been rejected. Although I now earn an adequate income as a free-lance lecturer and writer, and teach six months of each year at Stanford University, it seems evident to me that I have been blackballed from corporate employment. But I have no grounds for complaint, for who would hire a man who stole and later distributed his former employer's proprietary documents? I have accepted the termination of my engineering career as the price I must pay for bringing the EEI and Dragoumis documents before the public.

Despite the fact that I was fired from my job, that statutory immunities were denied me, and that I appear to have been blackballed from technical employment, I am very optimistic about the future. In the words of Department of Energy officials, the nuclear industry is "barely alive." (Since the disclosure of the Dragoumis memoranda, General Electric had difficulty selling reactor-containment systems featuring the Mark III design and suffered dozens of postponements and cancellations of earlier orders—including the two reactors ordered by PEPCO for the Douglas Point station.) Partly because of the Three Mile Island accident, a great many people are now skeptical of industry claims that the risks of nuclear power are minimal and that the benefits justify them. Every one of my 1974 allegations has been confirmed by other critics, several of whom have extensive industry and engineering experience. More important, the TMI accident validates many of these charges and bestows a degree of credibility on nuclear critics who for years endured harassment, reprisals, and pejorative labels by the pronuclear establishment. A close reading of the public statements and publications of these critics reveals a great deal of consistency. The interlocking nature of their charges is especially striking because they were made by engineers and scientists representing all three sectors—government, reactor vendors, and electric power companies—and who arrived at their conclusions independently.

The conflict of expert opinions on the matter of safety suggests that debate on this topic is unproductive and that a deeper issue is involved. Such has been suggested by Amory Lovins, a physicist and internationally recognized energy policy analyst, who comments on nuclear technology as follows:

> [U]ltimately its safety is limited not by our care, ingenuity, dedication or wealth . . . but by our inescapable human fallibility; limited not by our good intentions, but by gaps between intention and performance; limited not by our ability to solve problems on paper, but by our inability to translate paper solutions into real events. If this view were correct, it would follow that nuclear safety is not a mere engineering problem that can be solved by sufficient care, but rather a wholly new type of problem that can be solved only by infallible people. Infallible people are not now observable in the nuclear industry or in any other industry.

In this short analysis, Lovins pinpoints what I had dimly perceived—but very keenly felt—during my engineering career: that experts on each side of the nuclear issue disagree because they evaluate human experience in fundamentally different ways. The technological optimists—and I used to be one—are convinced that the major problems afflicting the nuclear industry are soluble and that technical fixes will play an important part in resolving these problems. They have faith in the perfectability of man, and it is a fair question whether this faith has an ideological or rational basis. They believe that a proper integration of humans and well-designed technical systems will compensate, with a generous margin of safety, for the unpredictable, unknown domains—the dark side of human potential that history documents and that technologists tend to dismiss as tractable. Technological skeptics, on the other hand, tend to reject these assumptions out of hand. But because the skeptical position is unlikely to support generous R&D subsidies and deployment of hazardous technologies, and because these are sought after as a means to achieve a growing gross national product, it is regarded by most Americans as faintly subversive until an event like the TMI accident convinces them that a healthy skepticism is their only protection against the hazards of proceeding too fast with imperfectly understood technologies.

Any analysis of the nuclear controversy tends to distill two issues that have occupied much of my time since 1974. The first turns on the question of how safe is safe enough? If nuclear systems have been designed as safely as engineers can make them, we must ask—and attempt to answer—whether this margin of safety is adequate, given the catastrophic effects of a major accident. The nuclear industry insists that the probability of such an accident is infinitesimal, and it is true that backup and redundant systems significantly reduce the chances of an accident. To some extent, these systems may buffer reactor operation from human error as well. But complex systems tend to malfunction for complex reasons and in ways undreamed of by their designers. In the end, it may be that man himself may govern accident probabilities that now appear favorably small because nuclear risks were calculated with primary attention to the *engineering* aspects, about which a great deal is known, rather than to the *human* aspects, about which there remains a great ocean of truth to be discovered.

The second issue concerns the division of labor and responsibility between engineers and executives. I believe that an engineer bears *major* responsibility for the safety of the system he designs, and *partial* responsibility for the way in which these systems are used. During the war years—and our country has faced three major wars in the last 35 years—certain pressures on engineers led to a condition where they abdicated more and more responsibility for safety and usage. These pressures, which carried over into peacetime, focused on getting a system operational as fast as possible. Because many of these systems were designed for direct use by or support of the military, engineers simply could not be bothered with the ethical problems inherent in the fact that their systems were being used to kill and maim soldiers and civilians. The issue turns on the fact that what should be the responsibility of the engineer is, to a major extent, co-opted by corporate executives interested in reducing ethical pressures on engineers in the interests of efficient production. After employing engineers, these executives set policy—more often than not by simply saying nothing—that communicates the idea to line employees that *broad questions of safety and usage are not their responsibility.* Certainly the penalty for disobeying this policy is underlined when an engineer takes matters into his own hands, asks sensitive questions in public, and is fired.

If most engineers have abdicated responsibility for these matters, and if executives have co-opted them, then it is also true that executives have not done a very satisfactory job of discharging these responsibilities. This has happened because the highest levels of most corporations are dominated by sales, marketing, and fiscal specialists rather than by senior engineers. The result is that engineering ethics, as I have defined them, play a small part in executive decisions, whether that decision is to market a reactor with unresolved safety problems or to put another on line when delays costs upwards of $400,000 per day. There have been many instances where management has made a fiscally unprofitable decision that favors public welfare, but these are infrequent and are the exceptions that prove the rule. It should not surprise anyone, then, that an occasional engineer upsets the applecart by assuming responsibility for executive matters that are, in his view, unsatisfactorily discharged. Most likely, he will feel keenly about these matters and decide that these responsibilities for safety and usage weigh upon him simply because no one else seems to be shouldering them. The whistle blower/exengineer later becomes interesting to citizens who start to ask who, if anyone, is in charge. At this point, the truly important questions are raised and the whistle blower's significance turns on issues of corporate responsibility rather than loyalty.

My experience has been that most engineers are honest, competent, and dedicated people who accept, as a matter of good manners, constraints on their freedom of speech and their right to question executive decisions. The fact that ethical considerations bear on these constraints does not occur to most of them. This oversight is partly the result of poor design of curricula at the undergraduate level, where courses on ethical problems are neglected in favor of additional, narrow training in specialized upper-division topics. Certainly, corporations have an interest in hiring people who defer questions of policy and broad responsibility to their superiors, and this may partly explain the curriculum defects. What I find most striking is that these executives are seldom the ones called upon to defend nuclear technology before the lay public, even though it is these executives who have lifted safety and usage responsibility from the consciences of line employees. Yet it is most often these line employees who appear in public, representing their company or profession, trying to defend a technology whose ethical implications they do not understand and the responsibility for which they are trying belatedly to recover.

How should the responsibility for safety and usage be shared among executives and engineers? If no one is willing to accept final responsibility, does it follow that everyone ends up sharing the responsibility equally and involuntarily? These questions have bothered me for years. They are important to me because the acts I have admitted to here and for which I have paid dearly derived from a unilateral assumption of responsibility for people I sensed were in danger. If these questions are seriously addressed, one answer emerges fairly easily: since executives are free from the detailed duties of engineering design, testing, and marketing, they should be the ones who have—or who should make—the time to deal with and discharge the responsibilities mentioned here. They are, after all, the leaders as well as the employers. This is not to vindicate the hundreds of thousands of engineers who choose to leave these questions to management. The point I would like to underline is that management must have been aware all these years that line engineers were acting obediently and unquestioningly, partly out of fear for their jobs, and that all line employees responded to these fears because management contrived constraints that created these fears in the first place.

So in the end I am inclined to pin responsibility for the engineer's gradual abdication of responsibility on his employers and, beyond them, on the network of managers and executives who developed and tolerated this abdication. This process occurred in the military and in industries other than nuclear power. But it was especially evident in the latter because so many line employees have come forward in the last ten years to criticize the industry. These employees had nothing to gain and everything to lose by blowing the whistle. And it was their employers who had the most to gain by listening; instead, they did everything in their power to convince the public that the whistle blowers were wrong.

The view of the industry that I now hold is that of an intensely bureaucratic, centralized, and dictatorial directorate of nuclear enthusiasts who used every possible means to deploy nuclear reactors worldwide as fast as possible. These executives and engineers avoided the underlying moral and ethical issues of nuclear power. They point to the irreversible deployment of nuclear reactors as grounds for dismissing vital issues as academic when raised, and for suppressing criticism of their objectives and tactics. My original suspicions of managerial incompetence have given way to an even less charitable view: Nuclear industry leaders dwell in the dark caves of the unconscious, and they scream when they see the light.

Additional Readings

Clinard, Marshall B. *Corporate Ethics and Crime: The Role of Middle Management.* Beverly Hills, Calif.: Sage, 1983.

Donaldson, Thomas. *Corporations and Morality.* Englewood Cliffs, N.J.: Prentice–Hall, 1982.

Glazer, Myron P. and M. Penina. "Whistleblowing." *Psychology Today* 20 (August 1986), pp. 37–43.

Heilbroner, Robert L. et al. *In the Name of Profit.* New York: Doubleday, 1972.

Kanter, Rosabeth Moss. *Men and Women of the Corporation.* New York: Basic Books, 1977.

Kanter, Rosabeth Moss and Barry A. Stein, eds. *Life in Organizations: Workplaces As People Experience Them.* New York: Basic Books, 1979.

Maccoby, Michael. "The Corporate Climber Has to Find His Heart." *The Big Business Reader: On Corporate America,* edited by Mark Green. New York: Pilgrim Press, 1983 rev. ed.

Margolis, Diane Rothbard. *The Managers: Corporate Life in America.* New York: Morrow, 1979.

Nader, Ralph, Peter J. Petkas, and Kate Blackwell, eds. *Whistle Blowing: The Report of the Conference on Professional Responsibility.* New York: Grossman, 1972.

Shorris, Earl. *Scenes from Corporate Life: Politics of Middle Management.* New York: Penguin Books, 1984.

Westin, Alan F., ed. *Whistle Blowing: Loyalty and Dissent in the Corporation.* New York: McGraw–Hill, 1981.

Epilogue:
Corporate Violence
and the Banality of Evil

IN 1941, I. G. Farben, the largest chemical company in Germany, began the construction of several massive plants at Auschwitz in order to produce synthetic rubber and fuel for the Nazi government. To build the facilities, Farben executives negotiated a labor contract with Heinrich Himmler whereby his Nazi S.S. (secret police) would provide an almost inexhaustible supply of slave labor from the nearby Auschwitz concentration camp (the infamous camp in which hundreds of thousands of Jews were systematically tortured and eventually exterminated). To maintain security and to punish the workers, the S.S. agreed to provide guards, or "bosses," mostly sadistic professional criminals, who frequently beat and tortured workers who could not keep up during the four-mile trip each day to and from the work site.[1]

With work proceeding slowly because of the workers' weakened condition, the Farben board of directors, in 1942, decided to set up their own labor concentration camp immediately adjacent to the factory site. Farben agreed to take over responsibility for the housing, feeding, and health of the slave-labor inmates. However, to profit handsomely from their $250 million corporate investment, the Farben board also adopted the principle that "all inmates must be fed, sheltered and treated in such a way as to exploit them to the highest possible extent, at the lowest conceivable degree of expenditure."[2] As part of the starvation diet of watery turnip soup provided all Auschwitz inmates, the Farben corporation added an extra ration of soup for its labor force, not out of concern for the health of the workers, "but to maintain a precisely calculated level of productivity."[3]

> The diet fed to I.G. Auschwitz inmates . . . resulted in an average weight loss for each individual of about six and a half to nine pounds a week. At the end of a month, the change in the prisoner's appearance was marked; at the end of two months, the inmates were

187

not recognizable except as caricatures formed of skin, bones, and practically no flesh.[4]

Between five and one hundred slave laborers died each day at the Farben factories with the life of the typical laborer estimated at three to four months. Workers too weak or sick to lift the steel girders and heavy cement construction blocks, which frequently outweighed them, were promptly marched off to the gas chambers. (Zyklon B, the commercial name of the lethal gas used in the gas chambers, also used for killing rodents and insects, was manufactured by a subsidiary of Farben and provided another source of lucrative profit for this corporate conglomerate, which had a 42.5 percent interest in the company.) Joseph Borkin describes the atrocities of Farben's labor policies when taken to their ultimate conclusion:

> By adopting the theory and practice of Nazi morality, [Farben] was able to depart from the conventional economics of slave labor in which slaves are traditionally treated as capital equipment to be maintained and serviced for optimum use and depreciated over a normal life span. Instead, I.G. reduced slave labor to a consumable raw material. . . . When no usable energy remained, the living dross [waste matter] was shipped to the gassing chambers and cremation furnaces . . . where the S.S. recycled it into the German war economy—gold teeth for the Reichsbank, hair for mattresses, and fat for soup.[5]

Of the approximately 300,000 workers who passed through the Farben plants on their way to the extermination centers at Auschwitz, at least 25,000 of these slave laborers were literally worked to death.

In addition to operating slave labor death camps, the Farben corporation arranged with the Nazi government to use 150 women inmates as medical guinea pigs in an experiment to produce a new sleep-inducing drug. Each of the women died in the experiment. A company letter to the Auschwitz concentration camp reveals the impersonal business attitude toward the experimental subjects:

> In contemplation of experiments with a new soporific drug, we would appreciate your procuring for us a number of women. . . . We received your answer but consider the price of 200 marks a woman excessive. We propose to pay not more than 170 marks a head. If agreeable, we will take possession of the women. We need approximately 150. . . . Received the order of 150 women. Despite their emaciated condition, they were found satisfactory. We shall keep you posted on developments concerning this experiment. . . . The tests were made. All subjects died. We shall contact you shortly in the subject of a new load.[6]

At the war crime trials in Nuremberg at the end of the war, the

Allies convicted and imprisoned twelve Farben executives for their part in the brutalization, murder, and enslavement of workers. (The prison sentences ranged from one and one-half to twelve years; however, the vast majority of persons directly involved in deployment and mistreatment of slave labor were never punished.) During the trial, the Farban defense attorney insisted that the executives of this giant international chemical firm were only doing what most business firms attempt to do—minimize labor costs and maximize profits. At the time, there were no laws forbidding the use of slave labor, and, the defense counsel argued, company officials would have been shot by the Nazi government if they refused to participate in the construction and operation of the synthetic rubber factories.

As part of the punishment of the convicted Farben executives, the Allies insisted that none of the executives be appointed to the boards of the three chemical companies (Hoechst, BASF, and Bayer) that were formed as the result of the forced break up of I. G. Farben. But once the control of the Allies had loosened, most of these Farben executives were quickly restored to their positions of managerial leadership in post-war Germany, and several of them were appointed to the boards of the newly established chemical companies. Upon release from prison, one of the top Farben officials was appointed to the supervisory board of the Hoechst company in 1955 and subsequently elected chairman; another key executive who had served seven years in prison became chairman of the Bayer company in 1956.

Although the I. G. Farben slave-labor atrocities are an extreme case, it suggests that persons often act differently in their organizational roles in large corporate bureaucracies than in their own private lives. Although respected members of the business community, these Farben executives were able to force some 25,000 laborers to work to death and to use women as subjects in lethal drug experiments. As Richard Rubenstein comments:

> The business of mass murder was both a highly complex and successful corporate venture. The men who carried out the business part of the venture were not uniformed thugs or hoodlums. They were highly competent, respectable corporate executives who were doing what they had been trained to do—run large corporations successfully. As long as their institutions functioned efficiently, they had no qualms whatsoever concerning the uses to which they were put.

The corporate mentality of the Farben conglomerate, while perhaps to some extent a wartime aberration, is not totally dissimilar to the attitude of impersonal economic rationality that seems to characterize many large corporations where there is often a moral *indifference* to the consequences of corporate lawbreaking. As Steven Box points out, "evil should not be unrecognized merely because it is as banal as indifference; indifference rather than intent may well be the greater cause of avoidable human suffering, particularly in the case of corporate crime."[8] Whether it be the sale of Tris laden pajamas to Third World nations, the refusal to inform workers of the deadly risks of inhaling cyanide fumes in the Film Recovery Systems factory, or the maintenance of cotton dust at levels that guarantee thousands of permanently disabled textile workers, large corporate enterprises seem to generate a pragmatic *amorality*—an ethical numbness.

How is it possible that men who are basically moral and decent in their own families—perhaps even generous in civic and charitable contributions—are able to engage in corporate acts that have extraordinarily inhumane consequences? The key to understanding this fundamental human enigma lies not in the pathology of evil individuals but in the culture and structure of large-scale bureaucratic organizations within a particular political economy. Thus, in addition to whatever else may be involved in explaining corporate violence, some insight may be provided by a brief examination of the organizational pressures and dilemmas that confront corporate executives in a capitalistic economy.

Goals, Priorities, and Pressures

Although large corporations may have other goals—enhanced prestige and power, increased market shares, product diversification into potentially competing industries, growth and stability, or other short-range goals—the long-run profitability of the corporation is ultimately the most basic and over-riding goal. "No matter how strongly managers prefer to pursue other objectives and no matter how difficult it is to find profit-maximizing strategies in a world of uncertainty and high information costs, failure to satisfy this criterion means ultimately that a firm will disappear from the economic scene."[9] In a capitalistic economy, profit-seeking firms must often compete in an uncertain and unpredictable environment. Competitive market pressures, fluctuating sales, increasing costs for safety and health measures, consumer and environmental concerns, government regulations, and other constraints may limit the ability of the business firm to achieve its profit goals through legitimate opportunities. Thus, some corporations may evade and violate the law or engage in practices that many Americans would consider unethical, endangering the well-being of workers, consumers, and citizens.

In response to the request of the Dupont corporation to use safety glass in the Chevrolet cars, Alfred P. Sloan, the former president of

General Motors, succinctly stated this corporate priority of profit—sometimes at any cost:

> I am trying to protect the interest of the stockholders of General Motors and the corporation's operating position—it is not my responsibility to sell safety glass. . . . You can say perhaps that I am selfish, but business is selfish. We are not a charitable institution—we are trying to make a profit for our stockholders.[10]

As the case of the Ford Pinto reveals, the automobile industry has not only been indifferent to pleas for greater auto safety, but in some instances has actively lobbied to prevent safety regulations that threatened corporate profits. From the rejection of safety glass and airbags to the refusal to redesign flawed gas tanks, the conviction that "safety doesn't sell" has needlessly destroyed human lives and caused crippling injuries.

For new employees joining a firm, the *internal organizational climate*—the corporate subculture—is not typically an environment suffused with ethical sensibilities and discussions of social responsibility. Instead, quantifiable performance criteria based on production goals, sales quotas, volume, costs, market shares, and quarterly profits pervade the corporate atmosphere. If socialized into a job routine that includes illegal or questionable ethical practices, the new job holder is apt to look for guidance from immediate superiors or peers and experiences pressures to "get on board and up to speed quickly."[11] Frequently, the illegal or unethical practices are so institutionalized that they simply appear to be part of the *normal* routine and are unreflected upon. Indeed, executives who are convicted of violating the law often react with surprise and shock that their actions were considered criminal or unethical by people outside the insulated occupational world of the corporation. One General Electric official, convicted for his part in the heavy electrical equipment conspiracy commented that price-fixing "had become so common and gone on for so many years that we lost sight of the fact that it was illegal."[12] As James Carey describes the attitudes of the pharmaceutical executives involved in the marketing of an anticholesterol drug with dangerous side effects: "No one involved expressed any strong repugnance or even opposition to selling the unsafe drug. Rather, they all seemed to drift into the activity without thinking a great deal about it."[13]

For the newcomer, subtle cues and shared corporate vocabularies ("he's a team player," "she's a producer," "he's on a fast track") clearly indicate the preferred role models and where the rewards lie. "Conversations about moral and ethical issues are almost doomed to be awkward, halting, and time-consuming to the point of painfulness"—and therefore unlikely to occur.[14] And powerful executive supervisors have many ways to keep conscience-troubled subordinates in line: the threat of demotion, transfer to a less desirable position, and subtle innuendo regarding the employee's abilities and future with the company.

Faced with the choice of refusing to follow orders and risking the stigma of organizational disloyalty, or "going along," many employees will reluctantly pursue the latter course. In a survey of 400 corporate managers in eighteen different industries, 50 percent of top-level and 84 percent of lower-level managers agreed to some degree with this statement: "Managers today feel under pressure to compromise personal standards to achieve company goals."[15] Two other surveys, one a random sample of corporate managers and the other a study of Uniroyal executives, found that between 64 and 70 percent of the managers perceived that their peers "would not refuse orders to market off-standard and possibly dangerous items" (although a majority of the managers said they would personally reject such orders).[16] John De Lorean, recalling his experiences as a former senior vice-president at General Motors commented on corporate pressures and the importance of being a "team player":

> There wasn't a man in top GM management who had anything to do with the Corvair who would purposely build a car that he knew would hurt or kill people.
> But, as part of a management team pushing for increased sales or profits, each gave his individual approval in a group to decisions which produced the car in the face of serious doubts that were raised about its safety, and then later sought to squelch information which might prove the car's deficiencies.[17]

Or consider the case of the NASA space shuttle, Challenger. On the frigid morning of January 28, 1986, the shuttle disintegrated minutes after lift-off, killing all seven astronauts. A presidential investigation revealed that despite numerous warnings by engineers for Morton Thiokol, Inc. that the solid rocket booster seals might prove defective at low temperatures, top management overruled their own engineers and gave approval for the ill-fated flight. Under strong pressure from a team of senior-level executives and NASA officials to make the shuttle launch—and procure the renewal of the lucrative $400 million solid booster contract at stake—the vice-president for engineering at Thiokol testified that he changed his position regarding the safety of the flight after being told "to shed his role as an engineer and take the role of a management person."[18] As the probe of the shuttle disaster deepened, evidence of a tangled web of NASA mismanagement, fraud, and corporate misconduct emerged revealing pressures to accommodate NASA launch schedules and enhance corporate profits that jeopardized the safety of the space shuttle program. (Government documents, for example, revealed that as early as 1980, Rockwell International, the prime contractor for the space shuttle, failed to report promptly to NASA defects in components of the space orbiter whose malfunction could threaten the Challenger or its crew. According to 1983 documents in the NASA Inspector General's office, officials at Jet Air, Inc., a subcontractor for Rockwell International, routinely falsified X-ray reports to conceal defective welds on the Challenger "to avoid the costs of rewelding.")[19]

For managers with a heavy stake in their position in the company, the moral trade-offs from corporate pressures to violate the law may sometimes cause severe discomfort. One laboratory supervisor, who was asked to go along with the cover-up of falsified test data on aircraft brakes to meet a deadline for a defense contract, explained:

> I've been an engineer for a long time, and I've always believed that ethics and integrity were every bit as important as theorems and formulas, and never once has anything happened to change my beliefs. Now this . . . Hell, I've got two sons I've got to put through school and I just . . .[20]

Another conspirator in the doctored test data commented on a similar dilemma:

> At forty-two, with seven children, I had decided that the Goodrich Company would probably be my "home" for the rest of my working life. The job paid well, it was pleasant and challenging, and the future looked reasonably bright. My wife and I had bought a home and we were ready to settle down into a comfortable, middle-age, middle-class rut. If I refused to take part in the . . . fraud, I would have to either resign or be fired.[21]

In the heavy-electrical-industry price-fixing conspiracy, the sentencing judge summarized the predicament of the participants:

> They were torn between conscience and an approved corporate policy, with the rewarding objective of promotion, comfortable security, and large salaries. They were the organization, or company man; the conformist who goes along with his superiors and finds balm for his conscience in additional comforts and security of his place in the corporate set-up.[22]

There is some empirical evidence that corporate managers who are shrewd and ambitious, men with "flexible moralities" and an eye on both the company's bottom line and their own career mobility, are likely to experience considerable success in today's executive suites. Indeed, as Edward Gross argues, high positions in corporate organizations seem to demand persons with such personal characteristics and "non-demanding moral codes": executives who can both sleep at night and make the cold, calculated decisions "for the good of the company." And it seems likely that after long years of service, such top-level executives gradually internalize the ideologies and goals of the company—and make them their own, as they profit personally from such goal attainment and organizational loyalty.[23]

Neutralizing Guilt

In view of the commitment of respectable corporate executives to the conventional social order, it is necessary for corporate officials who violate the law to neutralize the potential feelings of guilt and self-condemnation. There are many justifications and rationalizations that enable corporate functionaries to accomplish this social-psychological task and avoid any definition of themselves as criminal. Indeed, the very availability of these shared "vocabularies of rationalization" already existing within the corporate occupational culture is precisely what permits many managers to violate the law without any great burden of guilt or threat to their self-respect. The following mechanisms are some "techniques of neutralization" to help assuage one's conscience and rationalize criminal acts.[24]

Denial of Responsibility. A distinguishing characteristic of large-scale corporations is the fragmentation of responsibilities. In a hierarchial labyrinth of specialized tasks and segmented organizational units, employees can easily evade any sense of personal responsibility for the ultimate consequences of their actions. In the B.F. Goodrich scandal where the falsification of airplane test data jeopardized the safety of airplane pilots, officials who participated in the cover-up by falsifying data or by verbally approving the fraudulent reports repeatedly denied that their responsibility extended beyond that specific action. One test lab supervisor who "fudged" the data for the flawed aircraft brakes commented: "After all, we're just drawing some curves, and what happens to them after they leave here, well, we're not responsible for that."[25] Another supervisor, when confronted by a lab technician who demanded that the supervisor report the cover-up to the chief engineer of the plant, refused. When asked to justify his refusal, the supervisor replied: "Because it's none of my business, and it's none of yours. I learned a long time ago not to worry about things over which I had no control. I have no control over this." The lab technician persisted, however, appealing to the supervisor's conscience and pointing out that pilots might be killed or injured during flight tests if the brakes failed to hold. Becoming rather exasperated, the supervisor replied, "I just told you I have no control over this thing. Why should my conscience bother me?"[26]

In a bureaucratic organization, most employees see only a small part of the whole corporate enterprise and can conveniently ignore—or choose not to see—the larger implications of their occupational decisions. Bureaucracies *depersonalize*, and corporate officials rarely confront the victims whose faces are melted beyond recognition in fiery automobile crashes when defective gas tanks explode. It is unlikely that the senior executives at the Robins company who made the decision to keep the Dalkon Shield IUD on the market ever met any of the women who suffered from painful pelvic infections, or the mothers whose children were born retarded, or the women who lost their ovaries and can never have any children. One can only wonder what would have been the response of the executives who marketed thalidomide if they could have personally confronted some of the 8,000 children born with horrible deformities that this drug was suspected or producing. Would these officials have continued to "lie, suppress, bribe and distort" to keep this highly profitable, "non-toxic tranquilizer" on the market if they had come face to face with children such as Terry Wiles—"sixteen years old now but only two feet high, born without arms or legs, and with a protruding eye that had to be surgically removed—and . . . mothers ravaged by guilt . . .?"[27]

Decision-making must, to a large degree, be decentralized in mammoth corporations with multidivisional organizational structures (e.g., research and planning divisions, engineering departments, legal offices, production plants, sales and marketing divisions, corporate subsidiaries). Important operational decisions are made in a series of small steps at each organizational level in the corporate hierarchy, thereby diffusing responsibility. In this bureaucratic labyrinth, it is often difficult to find any specific individual at higher executive levels on whom to place the responsibility for short-cuts in product safety or distorted drug test results. Harried managers under pressure to achieve results may filter and edit information (e.g., questionable safety findings) before sending it up the corporate line of command to make their own department look good. Consequently, top company officials may sometimes have only partial information regarding what goes on at middle and lower levels of management.

Yet, to absolve themselves of any legal responsibility, upper-echelon executives may make it quite clear that they do not wish to be informed of all the sordid details used "to meet the competition" or "cope with the regulators," while they, at the same time, hold lower-level managers responsible for failure to meet production deadlines or profit quotas. Under excruciating pressure to meet extremely demanding goals, and aware that he or she can easily be replaced, the desperate manager, searching for a quick fix, can find illegal or unethical means attractive. In the heavy-electrical-equipment price-fixing conspiracy, top executives, after setting profit goals and market shares that virtually required price-fixing, made it quite clear to middle-level managers that they did not wish to learn of any illegal means that might be used to achieve these objectives.[29]

Denial of Injury. Another social-psychological device to avoid moral responsibility and alleviate feelings of guilt is to define what occurs as an unfortunate "accident" or the hazards inherent in dangerous work. None of the officials at the Ford Motor Company, at A. H. Robins, or at the Scotia Coal Company wished anyone to die or suffer from badly burned faces and managled limbs, or lose their reproductive organs. Managers can suppress medical data and reports of injuries or hazardous conditions and contend that they are acting in the best interest of their company. Speeding up production, taking shortcuts on product safety, falsifying lab tests, refusing to recall defective products or implement costly safety measures in the workplace—all are done, it can be rationalized, to enhance the company's profits. Although the consequences may be viewed as unfortunate, the insistence that there is no *intention* to harm (despite deliberate violations of safety and health regulations) takes the offender off the moral hook. Since the manager does not intend to hurt anyone, workers or consumers or the general public, such semantic sleight-of-hand conveniently insulates the company manager from realizing that his behavior is morally blameworthy, much less "criminal" (a view reinforced by the media stereotype of the criminal as the low-class predatory street offender).

In cases of work-related health problems (e.g., brown lung and asbestosis), company doctors and officials may argue that "more research is needed" to prove any link between the occurrence of cancer or other disabling ailments that may take years to develop, and the conditions existing in the textile and asbestos factories. That only a certain percentage of workers will develop the occupationally induced diseases, and the belief that those who do will be "compensated," helps blunt any sense of moral culpability from the failure to inform the workers at risk or to redesign a safer workplace. A former Johns-Manville medical director who developed the company policy of not informing asbestos workers that their routine physical examination revealed asbestosis explains his actions:

> Eventually, compensation will be paid to each of those men. But, as long as a man is not disabled it is felt he should not be told of his condition so that he can live and work in peace *and the company can benefit by his many years of experience.*[30]

Similarly, the difficulty in securing conclusive scientific evidence that chemical effluents contaminated groundwater used for drinking, and therefore caused an outbreak of cancer years later, helps to deflect any self-conception of company officials as criminally negligent. Between 1969 and 1986, twenty children in Woburn, Massachusetts, developed leukemia; eleven of them died. According to the U.S. Centers for Disease Control, the frequency of childhood leukemia in East Woburn, is seven times higher than expected on a chance basis.[31] Yet, even to win the case in a civil court, the parents of the dead children must prove a causal chain of events: that the companies were negligent in allowing dangerous chemicals to be disposed of in the soil; that these pollutants migrated to underground water supplies; and that the victims were exposed in sufficient quantities to cause cancer or death.

Denial of the Victim. One way to neutralize the moral implications of one's actions is to blame the victim for the harm. Corporate officials may insist that it was not any flaw in the intrauterine contraceptive device that caused the life-threatening pelvic infection, but the improper insertion of the IUD, or the lifestyles of "promiscuous women." Asbestos workers who develop lung cancer smoke too much and are predisposed to die from cancer anyway, "so why blame us?" A favorite argument in the automobile industry is that cars are not unsafe but road conditions and irresponsible drivers are the problem.

> It is an extraordinary experience to hear automotive "safety engineers" talk for hours without ever mentioning cars. They will advocate spending billions educating youngsters, punishing drunks and redesigning street signs. Listening to them, you can momentarily begin to think that it is easier to control 100 million drivers than a handful of manufacturers. They show movies about guardrail design and advocate the clear-cutting of trees 100 feet back from every highway in the nation. If a car is unsafe, they argue, it is because its owner doesn't drive properly. Or, perhaps, maintain it.[32]

Another way corporate officials can neutralize their guilt is to deny the victim full human status. In the Film Recovery Systems factory in Illinois, it was easier to force illegal hispanic or Polish aliens to handle a deadly cyanide solution without adequate safeguards, and consequently, jeopardize their lives. Anonymous victims, often of another race, from impoverished Third World nations—may help business managers avoid confronting their own qualms for dumping carcinogenic garments, dangerous drugs, highly toxic pesticides, or other products banned or under strict controls in this country. A recent report provides a vivid example of the risks involved in Central American countries where pesticide poisoning is a major problem among farmers and agricultural workers:

> A farm-supply store in Haiti is packed with multi-colored drums of pesticides—many of them banned in the United States. Clerks scoop

out the toxic white powders with their bare hands and put them into unlabeled plastic bags for sale to farmers on their crops. When the drums are empty, they are sold, unwashed, to peasants who use them as water containers."[1]

In response to the report, an official for Dow Chemical denied any moral responsibility for improper use of these exported pesticides (some so highly toxic that a teaspoon full of the chemicals can cause the death of an adult). "After a product has been removed to some banana plantation in Guatemala, you find it's difficult if not impossible to police and control its use."[35] Yet, no mention is made of how workers might become aware of the dangers involved when warning labels are printed in English or written in highly technical language, or, as occurs frequently with exports, warnings of the full extent of the dangers are glossed over or omitted entirely. As Robert Jackall points out, "In a world where the actual and symbolic interconnectedness of human action can be denied and where the faces of victims are unseen until it is too late, almost anything becomes permissible."[36] A University of California entomologist, who has studied the effects of toxic pesticides dumped in Central American countries, describes what may happen when agricultural workers are regarded as less than human:

The people who work in the fields are treated like half humans. . . . When an airplane flies over to spray, they can leave if they want, but they won't be paid their seven cents a day, or whatever. They often live in huts in the middle of the fields. Their homes, their children and their food get contaminated.[37]

Condemn the Condemners. A technique by which corporate officials may neutralize the moral bind of the law is to deny its legitimacy and to condemn not only it, but those government regulatory agencies that enforce such "unfair laws." In the 1980s, the campaign promise of "getting the government off our backs" symbolized the sanctity of the unfettered pursuit of profit in a "free-enterprise" system and the growing resistance to health, safety, and environmental regulations. Conservative business groups stepped up their attacks on the regulatory laws contending that they were oppressive, ambiguous, unnecessary, that they lowered profits and productivity, and in general, made it more difficult for American businesses to compete effectively in the world-wide economy. In 1983, a new senior administrator in the ideologically revamped Environmental Protection Agency, who had worked previously for a corporation under investigation for pollution violations, bitterly accused the EPA's own general counsel of overzealous enforcement and "alienating the primary constituents of this administration, the business community."[38]

In 1985, a chemical leak at the Union Carbide plant in Institute, West Virginia, hospitalized 135 workers. After an exhaustive investigation (partly prompted by international publicity of the gas leak in 1984 that killed 2,000 persons at the Carbide plant in Bhopal, India), the Occupational Safety and Health Administration imposed a $1.4 million fine on the company for over 200 violations of 55 federal safety and health laws. OSHA accused Union Carbide of willful and blatant disregard of the health and safety of its workers at the Institute plant. Among the alleged violations was the customary practice of asking workers to detect the presence of highly toxic phosgene gas by "sniffing the air after alarms indicated a leak." As Labor Secretary Brock sardonically commented: "They used to use canaries for that." (Phosgene, used in chemical warfare during World War I, is one of the most dangerous industrial gases; it causes lung damage and often results in death.) Angry at the magnitude of the proposed civil penalties and the adverse publicity, the president of Union Carbide lashed out at OSHA and condemned the agency as having "grossly distorted the actual safety conditions of the plant. Most of the citations are entirely unjustified."[39]

Appeal to Higher Loyalties. Finally, corporate managers may rationalize their evasions of laws and ethical constraints by appealing to a "morally superior" set of business ethics to justify their actions: the pursuit of profits in a free enterprise market economy unhampered by government interference. The belief in the moral superiority of this system of free enterprise—the provider of the nation's wealth and abundance, and the basis of human freedom and the American way of life—may release the manager from any feeling of moral obligation to comply with the law simply because it is merely a government regulation.[40] The only responsibility is to maximize profits for shareholders. And with a cultural legacy of "caveat emptor" (let the buyer beware) and a compensation insurance system for some work-related injuries, corporate management may refuse to recognize any further ethical responsibility for saving human lives and preventing harm. Conservative social critic and economist Milton Friedman has provided a strong ideological defense of this view of limited corporate social responsibility.

There is one and only one social responsibility of business—to use its resources and engage in activities designed to increase its profits so long as it stays within the rules of the game . . . [and] engages in open and free competition, without deception or fraud. . . . Few trends could so thoroughly undermine the very foundations of our free society as the acceptance by corporate officials of a social responsibility other than to make as much money for their stockholders as possible.[41]

If the only legitimate consideration is corporate profitability—with scant concern for ethical considerations—the use of cost-benefit analysis provides an impersonal and economically rational tool to help shape corporate decision-making. If voluntarily recalling millions of defective cars or deadly birth control devices, or lowering the level of cotton dust becomes too costly to the company—even if thousands of lives and much human suffering could be prevented—the executive may, with good conscience, reject such demands as not being "cost effective."

The company manager may also justify legal violations by appealing to another kind of higher morality. For instance, a factory manager may knowingly violate state or federal regulations on chemical dumping of pollutants or installation of expensive safety equipment, justifying these actions as necessary to keep corporate headquarters from closing the factory. Compliance with the law, the manager may contend, would make the plant unprofitable and make a ghost town of the community. Thus, "saving jobs" takes a higher ethical priority than obeying the law. One Texas political official commented on a federal investigation into the impact of asbestos on workers' health at the Pittsburgh-Corning plant in Tyler, Texas: "I think we are all willing to have a little bit of crud in our lungs and a full stomach rather than a whole lot of clean air and nothing to eat."[42] Eventually, the Tyler plant did close down, throwing hundreds of people out of work after an OHSA investigation found numerous safety violations. In recent years, many multinational corporations have tried to avoid such problems by relocating factories in foreign countries where labor costs are cheaper and there are no safety laws to erode corporate profits. As Raymond Michalowski points out, "rather than cease violations against worker health and safety, they have sought to locate new and less powerful victims."[43]

Controlling Corporate Violence, Whither America?

Many social critics have pointed out the massive difficulties in controlling corporate crime. Not only is it extremely hard to pinpoint individual responsibility in the complex maze of corporate bureaucracy, but the very evidence that would legally incriminate officials is often concealed within the corporation. The complexity of the task and the ability of corporate officials to thwart investigations often overwhelm enforcement agencies' limited resources. Beleaguered regulatory agencies find their legal powers eroded, their budgets slashed, and their enforcement efforts hampered by the intervention of politically connected, powerful corporate interests. Even when corporations are convicted, the use of administrative or civil courts and pleas of "nolo contendere" (no contest), largely removes the stigma of criminality. And since corporations cannot be imprisoned, the miniscule fines ("overhead business expenses") meted out to multibillion dollar companies hardly constitute a meaningful deterrent.

As the toll of human suffering from grave physical harms continues to rise, legal scholars and sociologists, in recent years, have proposed a variety of legal reforms to contain this wave of corporate violence. For example, a congressional committee in 1980 considered a proposal that would have required corporate managers who discover life-threatening safety and health hazards in the workplace or in a product to notify an appropriate federal agency or risk a $50,000 fine or two years in prison. After vigorous lobbying by manufacturers, the proposal died quietly in committee.

Indeed, there are innovative proposals to control corporate crime: e.g., requiring corporations convicted of crimes to advertise their injurious actions as both a form of punishment and consumer information; appointing public interest representatives on corporate boards to oversee court-mandated organizational and procedural reforms in the corporate decision-making process. From proposals for a civil "bill of rights" to protect and encourage whistle-blowers, to draconian criminal penalties such as "corporate capital punishment" (revoking the corporate charter or placing the "habitual criminal corporation" in federal receivership), social critics have made numerous proposals to make the criminal justice system more effective in controlling corporate crime.[44]

Yet, in the present political climate, these proposals, whatever their merit, stand little chance of implementation. Moreover, these kinds of legal reforms do nothing to change the basic economic forces in a capitalistic system that continue to generate pressures to use illegal or morally questionable means to achieve corporate goals. Few elected political officials in America seem willing to risk the economic dislocation that a radical attack on corporate criminality might precipitate. Only the most courageous legislators are apt to challenge the massive political power of corporations by writing effective laws. And even when a highly-publicized disaster goads reluctant lawmakers into advocating marginal legal reforms, especially in the crucial area of occupational safety and health, the power of corporations to weaken the laws with legal loopholes, to co-opt or otherwise render impotent the ability of governmental agencies to enforce new laws, all too often makes a mockery of this exercise in symbolic politics. Congressmen can reassure their constituents that they are safeguarding the public interest with this legal charade, but the ability of large corporations to continue to enhance their profits at the expense of human lives is likely to continue.

Despite such obstacles, pressures to control the antisocial acts of irresponsible corporations persist. During the last two decades, the Nader-inspired consumer protection movement, organized labor's demands for greater safety in the workplace, and the grass-roots efforts of angry families to save their communities from poisonous waste disposal have all helped to transform the individual victim's injury into an issue of public policy. Ultimately, however, a broad-based democratic political movement will be necessary to prevent further massive environmental destruction and human suffering caused by the practices of multinational corporations whose marketing and production facilities now span the entire globe. While incremental liberal reforms may save some lives and prevent some injuries, efforts that are valuable and should not be denigrated, such reforms are not easily won or sustained in the deregulatory conservative political climate of the present era. In the 1970s, new health and safety regulations, many of them now under attack, saved thousands of lives in factories, coal mines, and homes. Legal reforms led to a 50 percent reduction in crib deaths; a Consumer Product Safety Commission ruling requiring difficult-to-remove safety caps on pill bottles reduced emergency-room treatments for poisoning by 230,000 between 1973 and 1978 and prevented the deaths of 200 to 300 preschool children.[45]

Perhaps at this juncture in the American criminal justice system, a necessary and crucial step is to educate the public to the horrendous consequences of corporate wrongdoing—the damaged human lives, disease-stricken bodies, and other illnesses and injuries inflicted on workers and consumers. Until there is greater public understanding of the relationship between corporate decision-making and human suffering, indeed, until there is a public sensibility that provokes moral outrage at this corporate indifference, the far-reaching structural reforms that could make a major and lasting difference are unlikely to occur. Until more citizens perceive that assaulting a woman's body with a dangerously designed birth control device is as serious as assaulting her in the streets; that concealing the level of cotton dust particles is as unconscionable a crime as mugging an old man in an alleyway; that manufacturing and keeping on the market a defective car known to explode and burn on rear-end impact is as morally repugnant as any conventional form of criminal manslaughter—only when such acts are defined as "real crime," will further fundamental reform of the criminal justice system be possible.

The writings and research efforts of social scientists to foster this public awareness may lead to charges that such efforts are "biased." If such pejorative labels mean simply that sociologists are not indifferent to the outcome of what happens in their world, then most of us must plead guilty. As observers of social behavior, we can not avoid being morally involved in what we study. Nor are we any less biased by cloaking ourselves in a pseudo-scientific garb of "value-neutrality," assuming the posture of moral eunuchs. To be as objective as possible about our research data, to be aware of how our moral commitments shape our perceptions and conclusions, to be extremely clear about the criteria used to delineate crimes and make policy recommendations, all are imperative if we are to develop a more critical reflexivity toward our responsibilities as social researchers.[46] To pretend, however, that we are morally indifferent regarding the outcome of our research is to risk making our work sterile and socially irrelevant. And to refuse to make our values explicit, using instead the prevailing legalistic conceptions of crime, merely means that the value judgments provided by dominant political groups will continue to pervade the criminal justice system and distort public conceptions of the locus of harmful behavior in society.

Social scientists should not underestimate the difficulties of publicizing corporate violence in trying to change conceptions of criminality. Powerful political and economic interests strongly resist such reformulations of crime. It is the hope of a more humanistic criminology, however, that once a large part of the public broadens its conception of what constitutes criminal violence and begins to perceive more clearly the connections between callous decision-making in corporate bureaucracies and serious physical harms, more citizens will become actively involved in a political movement to bring about fundamental changes in the political economy and quality of American life.[47]

With such formidable obstacles to achieving major reforms, it is easy for sociologists to sink into a cynical mood of despair or detachment and withdraw into the politically safe study of conventional crimes of the poor and powerless. To retreat from a vigorous effort to expose corporate criminality in the face of these difficulties, however, leaves citizens not only with a myopic view of crime, but also ensures that such injurious corporate behavior will continue to erode the moral texture of the world in which our children shall grow up.

NOTES

1. This discussion of I. G. Farben is based on the writings of Joseph Borkin, *The Crime and Punishment of I. G. Farben* (New York: Free Press, 1978); Richard L. Rubenstein, *The Cunning of History* (New York: Harper & Row, 1978), chap. 4; David R. Simon and D. Stanley Eitzen, *Elite Deviance*, 2d ed. (Boston: Allyn and Bacon, 1986), pp. 227–228.

2. Borkin, p. 121.

3. Rubenstein, p. 58.

4. Borkin, p. 125.

5. Ibid., p. 126.

6. John Braithwaite. *Corporate Crime in the Pharmaceutical Industry* (London: Routledge & Kegan Paul, 1984), p. 5.

7. Rubenstein, pp. 62–63.

8. Steven Box. *Power, Crime, and Mystification.* (London: Tavistock, 1983), p. 21.

9. F. M. Scherer, quoted in Marshall B. Clinard. *Corporate Ethics and Crime.* (Beverly Hills, Calif.: Sage, 1983), p. 18.

10. Quoted in James W. Coleman, *The Criminal Elite.* (New York: St. Martin's Press, 1985), p. 40.

11. James A. Waters. "Catch 20.5: Corporate Morality as an Organizational Phenomenon." *Organizational Dynamics* (Spring 1978), p. 6.

12. Quoted in Gilbert Geis, "The Heavy Electrical Equipment Antitrust Cases of 1961." In *White Collar Crime,* edited by Gilbert Geis and Robert F. Meir. (New York: Free Press, 1977, rev. ed.), p. 123.

13. James T. Carey. *Introduction to Criminology.* (Englewood Cliffs, N.J.: Prentice–Hall, 1978), p. 384.

14. Waters, p. 10.

15. Archie B. Carroll. "Managerial Ethics: a Post–Watergate View." *Business Horizons* (April 1975), p. 77.

16. Carl Madden, quoted in Marshall B. Clinard and Peter C. Yeager. *Corporate Crime.* (New York: Free Press, 1980), p. 67.

17. Quoted in Mark Green and John F. Berry. *The Challenge of Hidden Profits.* (New York: Morrow, 1985), pp. 270–271.

18. Philip M. Boffey. "Rocket Engineers Tell of Pressure for a Launching." *The New York Times,* 26 February 1986, p. B–7. See also "Pointing Fingers." *Newsweek,* 10 March 1986, p. 40.

19. Stuart Diamond, "NASA Cut or Delayed Safety Spending," *The New York Times,* 24 April 1986, p. B–4.

20. Kermit Vandivier. "Why Should My Conscience Bother Me?" In *In the Name of Profit,* by Robert L. Heilbroner et al. (New York: Doubleday, 1972), p. 22.

21. Ibid., p. 24.

22. Geis, in Geis and Meier, p. 125.

23. Edward Gross. "Organizational Crime: A Theoretical Perspective." In *Studies in Symbolic Interaction,* edited by Norman K. Denzin, vol. 1. (Greenwich, Conn.: Jai Press, 1978), pp. 67–72; Box, pp. 38–43.

24. Gresham M. Sykes and David Matza. "Techniques of Neutralization: A Theory of Delinquency." *American Sociological Review* 22 (December 1957), pp. 667–70; Michael L. Benson. "Denying the Guilty Mind: Accounting for Involvement in a White-Collar Crime." *Criminology* 23 (November 1985), pp. 583–607.

25. Vandivier, p. 22.

26. Ibid., pp. 23–24.

27. Robert Jackall. "Crime in the Suites." *Contemporary Sociology* 9 (May 1980), p. 357.

28. John C. Coffee, Jr. " 'No Soul to Damn: No Body to Kick': An Unscanda-

lized Inquiry into the Problems of Corporate Punishment." *Michigan Law Review* 79 (January 1981), pp. 397–400; Clinard, pp. 95–102; George Getschow. "Some Middle Managers Cut Corners to Achieve High Corporate Goals." *The Wall Street Journal*, 8 November 1979, p. 1.

29. See Geis, "The Heavy Electrical Equipment Antitrust Cases of 1961."

30. M. David Ermann and Richard J. Lundman. *Corporate Deviance.* (New York: Holt, Rinehart and Winston, 1982), p. 73.

31. "Water Pollution Trial Against 2 Corporations Opens in Massachusetts." *Syracuse Post-Dispatch*, 11 March 1986, p. 8; "Why Business Is Watching This Pollution Case." *Business Week*, 24 March 1986, p. 39.

32. Mark Dowie. "Pinto Madness." *Mother Jones* (September/October 1977), p. 24.

33. Nancy Frank. *Crimes Against Health and Safety.* (New York: Harrow and Heston, 1985), p. 55.

34. Quoted in ibid., p. 47.

35. Ibid.

36. Jackall, p. 356.

37. Quoted in David Weir, with Mark Schapiro and Terry Jacobs. "The Boomerang Crime." *Mother Jones* (November 1979), p. 42.

38. "Mrs. Gorsuch Pollutes the E.P.A." *The New York Times*, 16 February 1983, p. A–30.

39. All quotes in this paragraph from Kenneth B. Noble. "Union Carbide Faces Fine of $1.4 Million on Safety Violations," *The New York Times*, 2 April 1986, pp. A–1, A–15.

40. Box, p. 57.

41. Quoted in Simon and Eitzen, p. 239.

42. Quoted in Raymond J. Michalowski. *Order, Law, and Crime.* (New York: Random House, 1985), p. 334.

43. Ibid. See also Barry I. Castleman. "The Double Standard in Industrial Hazards." *Multinational Monitor* (September 1984), pp. 4–8.

44. See John Braithwaite and Gilbert Geis. "On Theory and Action for Corporate Crime Control." *Crime and Delinquency* 27 (April 1982), pp. 292–314; Christopher D. Stone. *Where the Law Ends: The Social Control of Corporate Behavior.* (New York: Harper & Row, 1975); Ermann and Lundman, pp. 131–75.

45. Mark Green and Norman Waitzman. *Business War on the Law.* rev. 2d ed. (Washington, D.C.: The Corporate Accountability Research Group, 1981), p. 157; John Braithwaite. "White Collar Crime." Edited by Ralph H. Turner and James F. Short, Jr. *Annual Review of Sociology* 11, (Palo Alto, Calif.: Annual Reviews Inc., 1985), pp. 15–16; David Bollier and Joan Claybrook. *Freedom from Harm: The Civilizing Influence of Health, Safety, and Environmental Regulation.* (Washington, D.C. and New York: The Public Citizen and Democracy Project, 1986).

46. Ronald Kramer. "Studying Crime Where There Is No Law: Corporate Crime in the Multinational Context." (unpublished paper presented at the American Society of Criminology (November 1984, revised February 1985). See also Ronald C. Kramer. "Defining the Concept of Crime: A Humanistic Perspective." *Journal of Sociology and Social Welfare* 12 (September 1985), pp. 469–87.

47. See Simon and Eitzen, pp. 251–71; Martin Carnoy and Derek Schearer. *Economic Democracy: The Challenge of the 1980's.* (Armonk, N.Y.: M.E. Sharpe, 1980); Michael Harrington. *Decade of Decision: The Crisis of the American System.* (New York: Simon and Schuster, 1980); Samuel Bowles, David M. Gordon, and Thomas E. Weisskopf. *Beyond the Waste Land: A Democratic Alternative to Economic Decline.* (Garden City, N.Y.: Doubleday/Anchor, 1984).

Index

207

51 059